PRAISE FOR

# Wild Feminine

"Never before have I seen an author put into words concepts that encompass the deepest spiritual meaning and eternal symbolism of what it means to be a woman. Kent's book is a must-read for any student or teacher of the mysteries of the female body and the energies that define us."

—**Rosita Arvigo, DN**, traditional healer and founder of the Arvigo Techniques of Maya Abdominal Massage, author of *Sastun*, *Spiritual Bathing*, and *Rainforest Remedies*

"By suggesting a return to the root, Tami Lynn Kent offers direction for a path largely forgotten. Within the pages of *Wild Feminine* lies great hope for women, natural birth, and all things precious to the female body."

—**Ina May Gaskin**, midwife and author of *Spiritual Midwifery* and *Ina May's Guide to Childbirth*

"As a former midwife and the current organizer of international conferences for women, I am thrilled to recommend this unique book by Tami Lynn Kent. There is not a woman in the world who would not benefit from reading it. Whether you are seeking healing from emotional or sexual wounding or you just want to learn how to more fully enjoy and inhabit the most feminine aspect of yourself, this book will be a friend for life."

—**Elizabeth Lesser**, cofounder of Omega Institute, author of *The Seeker's Guide* and *Broken Open*

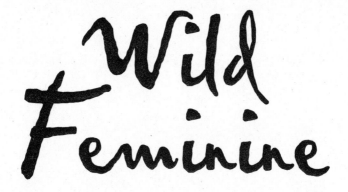

# Wild Feminine

## Finding Power, Spirit & Joy
## in the Female Body

# Tami Lynn Kent

**ATRIA** PAPERBACK
New York London Toronto Sydney

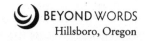

BEYOND WORDS
Hillsboro, Oregon

ATRIA BOOKS

A Division of Simon & Schuster, Inc.
1230 Avenue of the Americas
New York, NY 10020

BEYOND WORDS

20827 N.W. Cornell Road, Suite 500
Hillsboro, Oregon 97124-9808
503-531-8700 / 503-531-8773 fax
www.beyondword.com

The information contained in this book is intended to be educational and not for diagnosis,
prescription, or treatment of any health disorder whatsoever. This information should not
replace consultation with a competent healthcare professional. The content of this book
is intended to be used as an adjunct to a rational and responsible healthcare program
prescribed by a professional healthcare practitioner. The author and publisher are in no
way liable for any misuse of the material.

Managing editor: Lindsay S. Brown
Editor: Jenefer Angell
Copyeditor: Ali McCart
Proofreader: Gretchen Stelter
Design: Devon Smith
Composition: William H. Brunson Typography Services
Cover Art © 2008 Susan Gross, www.susangross.com
Author Photo: Shayne Berry, www.shayneberry.com

First Atria Paperback/Beyond Words trade paperback edition February 2011

**ATRIA** BOOKS and colophon are trademarks of Simon & Schuster, Inc.
Beyond Words Publishing is a division of Simon & Schuster, Inc.

For more information about special discounts for bulk purchases,
please contact Simon & Schuster Special Sales at 1-866-506-1949 or
business@simonandschuster.com.

The Simon & Schuster Speakers Bureau can bring authors to your live event.
For more information or to book an event, contact the Simon & Schuster Speakers
Bureau at 1-866-248-3049 or visit our website at www.simonspeakers.com.

Manufactured in the United States of America

30  29  28  27  26  25  24  23  22  21

*Library of Congress Cataloging-in-Publication Data*

Kent, Tami Lynn.
    Wild feminine : finding power, spirit & joy in the female body / Tami Lynn Kent.
        p.   cm.
    1. Mind and body.   2. Femininity.   I. Title.
    BF161.K47 2011
    155.3'33—dc22

                                                            2010035265

ISBN: 978-1-58270-284-1
ISBN: 978-1-4516-1021-5 (ebook)

The corporate mission of Beyond Words Publishing, Inc.: *Inspire to Integrity*

# CONTENTS

*Dear Reader,*

*I invite you to journey deep into the heart of your female body, to your root place, and to the root of all womanhood. Discover this landscape of the wild feminine. Find the connection between creative energy flow and the core of your body to reclaim the radiance that is rightfully yours.*

*The stories in this book reflect my work with women to offer guidance and awareness for the potential within our pelvic bowl and our feminine energy. Each story is a composite created to honor the true essence of healing I've witnessed while also protecting the privacy of those women who have graced my work. You do not need a practitioner to make profound shifts in your body and life; it is my intention that this book, distilled from the collective wisdom of the female body, will assist you.*

*This book is not meant to take the place of medical advice or your own intuition.*

*May you and your body be blessed.*

*The Great Work that is beginning is the realization of the feminine as the bridge between God and humankind.*

—Marion Woodman
*Bone: Dying into Life*

*The female body may represent one of feminism's least-touched frontiers, perhaps one of its final frontiers.*

—Caroline Knapp
*Appetites: Why Women Want*

# Foreword

Life in the twenty-first century presents new and unprecedented challenges for women. Major social changes, including those won by feminism, have given modern women an entrée into public life that would have been unthinkable for our female precursors, remembering that American women only received the right to vote in 1920. This inclusion as card-carrying citizens in a masculine world, although a welcome and just development, has created specific issues that our foremothers, whose world was overwhelmingly feminine, did not have to face.

For example, how do we, working in an office, factory, or other institution, accommodate the changes in our bodies and minds that accompany our monthly cycles? How can we ensure that our working conditions will not harm the babies we gestate? Is it possible to work apart from our infants and maintain our breastfeeding relationship? Do we continue paid employment while our children are young, and if so, how can we make the best provision for our children and their real needs for our loving care? How do we keep our public face as we make the transition through menopause, a passage that so often demands that we withdraw to complete our inner work?

These examples highlight the conflicts many women face as we balance our presence in the masculine world with our feminine needs and concerns. One response—perhaps the most rewarded in our culture—is to deny our female bodies: to adopt a pseudo-masculine approach that minimizes our bodies' innate feminine functions. Society sanctions this attitude and provides the means for menstrual concealment and suppression, birth interventions that override the body's natural process, separation of mothers and babies, formula feeding, and the treatment of menopause with hormonal substances, among others.

While each of these may be convenient at the time (and easier choices, culturally, than choosing menstrual retreat, natural birth, breastfeeding, mother-baby dependency, and unmedicated menopause), there is a downside. Each time we deny our female functions, each time we deviate from our bodies' natural path, we move farther away from our feminine roots. This can create distress within our bodies and can set the scene for further problems, physically and emotionally, for ourselves and our families.

For example, social pressures against breastfeeding (and other intimate forms of mother-baby contact) and the widespread promotion of nonhuman milk for human babies have resulted in a generation of mothers and babies who were denied the specific and evolutionary goodness of breastfeeding. Researchers are now linking our current epidemics of heart disease, high blood pressure, obesity, breast cancer, and childhood diabetes with this mass deprivation of feminine function. Similarly, recent research is highlighting that hormonal medications used to suppress menopause may increase the risks of breast cancer and heart disease: conditions that hormones were initially touted as preventing.

There is good news, however: no matter how strong the denial or how often we have turned away, our female bodies have not forgotten their functions. Our bodies are hardwired with this deep knowing and will call us back to reclaim the feminine for ourselves, in our own particular and specific way. And often it is our suffering in these especially female areas—menstruation, sexuality, abortion, miscarriage, birth, mothering, menopause, for example—that sets us on the path to healing our inner feminine.

*Healing* literally means "to make whole," and this wholeness is unique for each of us. Therefore, there is no fixed agenda, no stereotype of femininity except authenticity and joy, for our bodies are also the source of pleasure and fulfillment, whether through lovemaking, ecstatic birth, or the sensual pleasures of breastfeeding. Even menstruation can be immensely pleasurable, given time and space.

This is the truth so beautifully articulated in *Wild Feminine*: that our female bodies need us now more than ever, and that we too need the wisdom, the wildness, the passion, the joy, the vitality, and the authenticity that we can gain through this most intimate of reconciliations.

Tami Lynn Kent gives us more than a message: she also provides practical tools to reclaim our original female power and passion. This book contains an energetic map of the feminine landscape: that which is contained within our pelvic bowl. Through exploring and reconnecting with this terrain, a process that she calls Holistic Pelvic Care, Tami offers us a path back to the root of our femininity—a coming home to what is truly ours, as we rediscover our own feminine energy. This is mind-body medicine at its best and most sacred.

*Wild Feminine* also offers activities, reflections, and rituals that can help us understand and integrate our female experiences, and be compassionate with ourselves. Like a wise teacher or friend, this book encourages us to inhabit our wholeness, to find our direction, to release our restrictions, and to bring an ongoing awareness to our lives. Tami Lynn Kent weaves her feminine wisdom through the text so we emerge with more understanding of our inner feminine and our female cycles: our monthly ovulation-menstruation cycle and the larger cycle that moves from menstruation, pregnancy, child-birth, and breastfeeding back to menstruation.

Life in the twenty-first century may be challenging for women, but we are blessed with a growing collection of resources to guide us. *Wild Feminine* offers wisdom and guidance that has the potential to heal the feminine in each of us and in our culture.

—Sarah J. Buckley, MD
Sarah is a family physician, mother of four,
and author of *Gentle Birth, Gentle Mothering*
www.sarahjbuckley.com

# Reclaiming the Wild

I am drumming. Twenty women form a circle on the floor. They lie with heads together and legs extended, each pointing out from the center like a great star that pulsates with the beat of this drum. I ask the women to feel the drum's vibration in the root of their bodies. They follow the drumbeat to their wombs, where life itself begins.

Encircled by pelvic bones round and smooth, the root of the female body is like a bowl. Here, in her womb, a woman will find the energy she holds for herself and for mothering her creations. For centuries, women have been the bowl- and basket-makers, weaving containers that held food or water just as their bodies held the energy of the children and home. In urban settings and modern times, female roles have been redefined. But a woman's body still holds or releases energy from her root place, just as it always has.

Women are the energy keepers, their bodies a record of past events. As a woman travels to the root of her body, to her pelvic bowl where she stores this accumulated energy, she discovers what she has been given—and makes her way forward from there.

The drumming stops. Rising from the floor, each woman rights herself to sitting. They look at one another, wearing the face of the wild. They have journeyed into the source of their womanhood. Remembering long-forgotten landscapes, women speak of ancestors, ancient songs, births, and spirits: the terrain of the wild feminine. A communal spring of distilled beauty, the wild feminine revives each one. Breath upon breath, they are calling her back, retracing her path in their roots, reclaiming the wild in themselves.

# Coming Home

*I* did not begin my work in women's health looking for the wild feminine; the wild feminine found me. I was unaware of her absence until I sat with woman after woman who was profoundly disconnected from the root of her body, this physical place which houses the pelvic organs and channels the creative flow.

With my mother's passion for dance imprinted in my cells, I have always seen the body as a vehicle for expression. I found my way to physical therapy through the joy I experience in walking, playing sports, doing yoga—simply moving my body. My active sons would be surprised, they have seen me so often in a slower, pregnant form or sitting to nurse a baby. But movement inspired my work with the body.

Though it was my dream to work in women's health, I considered attending medical school because I had never heard of women's health as its own field of physical medicine. A fascination with movement patterns and how they influence the body directed me to physical therapy, but I rediscovered women's health in the third year of my graduate program. A guest speaker came to share her practice of physical therapy specifically for women. As she spoke, I knew the combination of physical therapy and women's healthcare was my true calling.

When I established my practice as a women's health physical therapist, in the outpatient clinic of a large hospital, my clients were typically beyond menopause and experiencing severe pelvic symptoms. Women came by referral from a urologist, and my treatment techniques were often a last resort prior to pelvic surgery for bladder leakage or uterine prolapse (when the uterus falls toward the vaginal opening). Pelvic surgery is not inevitable but may become necessary after the long-term effects of pelvic imbalance. Pelvic imbalance can also cause women to suffer needlessly from back or pelvic pain, decreased libido, and diminished vitality. Living with prolonged pelvic imbalance, a woman further loses touch with her creative center. Working with my clients' bodies, I felt the great weight of their unspoken grief regarding this loss; but at the time, I did not recognize its source in the unaddressed imbalances in their core.

Only after birthing my first son and nursing my own vagina through postpartum healing did I find that I too was estranged from my root. Taking care of my pelvic bowl for the first time, I encountered a well of emotions regarding my long-forgotten feminine needs. To identify and then address these feminine needs—for living in a sustainable manner, giving form to my creative energy, and receiving daily nourishment—I traversed the far reaches of my feminine terrain. I learned to weave my own way of making a joyful life, giving birth to two more sons, tapping into a deeper source to nurture myself, my creative life, and my children.

## Integrative Pelvic Care

The experience of connecting with my own root led me to reinvent my practice of women's health. I left the hospital clinic and opened an office in a more intimate homelike setting and began to offer preventive and postpartum pelvic care. I also developed an integrative practice I call Holistic Pelvic Care™, which incorporates a range of healing practices to restore balance in a woman's pelvis. Even traditional Western medicine acknowledges the benefits of recognizing connections between mind, body, and spirit; yet women's pelvic health has not generally been associated with this holistic approach. Holistic Pelvic Care combines the physical medicine practices of vaginal massage and organ alignment techniques with visualization and body awareness exercises to restore physical balance and energetic flow in a woman's pelvic bowl.

Without integrative pelvic care, I realized, most women simply learn to live with the pelvic imbalances resulting from childbirth, accumulated stress, or other events. Even beyond treating chronic pelvic symptoms, pelvic care ought to be an essential component of women's health. Today's women have chronic core tension due to a lack of awareness of pelvic wellness, habits—like prolonged sitting—that maintain pelvic stagnation, and a general disconnect from the feminine. Women benefit from forming an internal knowledge of their own feminine range, and ultimately rebuilding the underlying patterns limiting their core vibrancy and self-expression. By caring for the root of the female body as part of basic healthcare, and with a holistic perspective, we can address and heal both obvious and subtle imbalances, reversing the predominant trend of disregard for women's pelvic needs.

As my practice has grown, women have come to my office to heal themselves from birthing or to simply reconnect with the root, and then they often tell their friends to come. Though my clients are now typically younger or holistically minded, and presumably part of a more progressive population, each woman discovers that she has traveled a number of years without really knowing her root. I continue to witness a universal pelvic disconnect. Sometimes the detachment is physical: a woman has difficulty feeling her vaginal muscles. Other times it is emotional: a woman disassociates herself from her pelvic space as a way of coping with painful associations regarding femininity or her body. More subtly, this pelvic disconnect is energetic. Women experience diminished energy in the pelvic bowl because they do not regularly or consciously utilize their core creative capacity; they do not know how to cultivate feminine energy in their bodies.

Physical medicine is my art, and working in the root of the female body is like making sculpture; it requires the practitioner to attune to the deeper currents that give shape to a physical structure. Reading the physical patterns in the pelvis and restoring the vital energy flow are skills honed by respectfully listening to the body's wisdom. Skilled hands are a blessing because, for most women, the root has scarcely been approached with the reverence it deserves. My hands and my heart have sat with many women, and I have come to respect the creative capacity carried in the female body.

## The Link between Physical and Energetic

The physical process of realigning a woman's pelvic muscles eventually led me to a contemplation of how we as women embody our womanhood, an exploration of the ways the body records what it means to be female. Sitting at the root and listening to women's stories, I began to notice how root energy patterns were related to a woman's creative essence and how these patterns governed her usage of creative energy in everyday life. I took notes on these patterns, piecing them together to identify greater themes.

Energy is the fuel for our cells, giving life to our bodies and empowering our ability to create a robust and fulfilling existence. Energy flows in the body like river currents. The physical body interacts with the energy flow much like a riverbed channels and responds to the flow of the water. By understanding the connection between the patterns in our physical bodies and the resulting direction of creative energy flow into various aspects of our lives, we can strengthen those patterns that are beneficial and change the patterns that limit our true potential.

In my work with women, I find that just as physical patterns in the body can be changed in beneficial ways, the energy patterns of the pelvic bowl can be identified and transformed so that a woman may consciously direct her creative abilities. With the creative seeds of the ovaries and the gestational ability of the womb, the female body contains unlimited creative potential (the energy potential remains even if the organs have been removed). When a woman knows how to access her root place, she finds the energy for building her creative dreams, nurturing her creations, and changing the core patterns that diminish her radiance. She explores the link between physical form and energy flow and communes in the realm of the wild feminine.

## The Return of the Feminine

What began as a notebook of case studies documenting the healing I witnessed in the female body eventually became *Wild Feminine*. This book is a guide for exploring the vibrant feminine ground which women may come to understand and reclaim. *Wild Feminine* gives voice to an emerging women's movement: women of all ages and backgrounds are returning to the female body, reclaiming the creative force that arises from our center, and discovering its potential in daily life. A woman's root is her best resource for creating and integrating an empowered expression of the feminine.

The terms *divine*, *sacred*, and *spirit* will be used throughout this book. I am not writing from a religious point of view, although a woman may connect with the spiritual feminine realm in the practice of her own religion. Rather, I am addressing the individual experience of living each day with spirit. Living in relationship to spirit is a uniquely personal journey. It means awakening to the sacredness in every moment and all forms of life.

Wherever there is an absence of power, spirit, or joy in a woman's life, she has lost touch with her wild self. Each feminine loss is registered in the root of the female body, and to the body a woman must return in order to retrieve the full expression of her own wild feminine.

Though I do explore the energy of both the masculine and the feminine, the content of this book focuses on the feminine because it is imperative that women especially begin to recognize and reclaim the feminine in themselves. As the energy keepers and the ones who gestate life for our communities, we must learn how to restore the feminine energy flow in our bodies. When the feminine returns to the female body, the masculine is naturally inspired to reinvent the outer structures (roles, relations, work, home) in a more sustainable and life-giving manner. Natural systems are self-regulating once the core balance is restored.

Additionally, our creative lives are in the process of transformation. In the past fifty years, with the advent of birth control and professional career options, women are having fewer or no children. In just two or three generations, women have gone from having an average of six or eight children to just one or two. As a result, women have many more menstrual cycles during their fertile years and, with the widespread use of menstrual products, have increasingly been able to move at a continuously fast pace, with less regard for their bodily cycles. Often because of delayed childbearing choices, women are having difficulty conceiving or sustaining full-term pregnancies. Though our fertility cycles have evolved over thousands of years, the recent changes in our bodily experience of fertility have far outpaced evolution. The rhythms of our bodies are still linked to our women ancestors whose creative potential was typically expressed through carrying, birthing, and mothering children.

As a women's health physical therapist who spends many hours working on the pelvic bowl, I recognize that the very advantages of creative freedom, such as an abundance of professional opportunities and birth control options for women, have also taken us outside of our creative centers. Witnessing women reconnect with their bodies, I have seen that the body often reflects a more maternal, home- or earth-based essence. Yet, even as we transform our lives as women, the pelvic bowl has resources to assist us. To return to our bodies, we do not need to take a step backward but rather simply apply the creative energy we already carry to our present situation.

Because the creative flow in our bodies has evolved over time through pregnancy and birthing, it is helpful to reflect on these physical processes (as well as to examine ovulation, menstruation, miscarriage, and menopause) to learn about our creative energy. My hope is that whether or not you have had children, and regardless of whether you are still menstruating, you will read each story within *Wild Feminine* for the deeper patterns and clues that may reveal how to engage with your own creative essence. These physical processes provide insight for the creative cycles that run throughout our lives; it is worth returning to our origins in order to comprehend the essential feminine resources in the root.

## A Vast Potential Within

Your creative essence is a powerful current that flows through you. Rather than shaping or defining your creative energy by external factors (careers, partners, children, past experiences, and so on), you can work with the creative flow directly in your center. Focusing on this, you recognize the vast potential within—a whole range of energy resources and guidance from the wisdom of the body and the inner connection to spirit—and that we typically only access a small part of this landscape. Rather than realizing the full capacity of our creative core, we accept the limitations (ways of holding ourselves back or shutting down our creative energy) that we have inherited or formed in reaction to wounds or certain roles, and as a result, we diminish our natural abilities to receive true healing, new resources, vital energy, or unclaimed ground.

*Wild Feminine* will teach you how to work with the physical structure of your root and tap into the concentrated organ energies to change your relationship with the energy you draw from the environment and the greater spiritual realm. Through stories and guided exercises, you will find the energetic and physical connections to a whole creative range in the root of your body. These connections will allow you first to examine what is there and then to begin to trust and use the potential of your root in daily life.

In the first chapter, I introduce the language I developed to describe my observations from working with clients and also cultivating my own wild femininity. Chapter 2 teaches how to read the physical patterns of your pelvic bowl, how to do vaginal massage, and how your body patterns influence your creative flow. Chapter 3 describes how to dismantle restrictive feminine identities and renew your feminine spirit. The emotional energies of shame, sadness, grief, fear, rage, and joy are addressed in subsequent chapters. These emotions are often encountered when tapping into the energy of the pelvic bowl. Rather than stored or held, emotional energy is meant to move and activate your awareness; each emotion has a distinct purpose in restoring your feminine range.

Read about ovarian and uterine energies in chapters 4 and 5 to learn about the energetic capacity of your female body and how to clarify the energy in your bowl. Chapter 6 reveals how your feminine range expands when the energy of your lineage wounds, and other defining lines, are transformed. Chapter 7 shares the joy of making and applying your own root medicine in daily life, and each chapter contains exercises to take care of your root and cultivate the relationship between the physical and energetic to give intentional form to your creative expression.

The appendix contains information for starting a *Wild Feminine* Book Club. This section provides suggestions for using the material in this book to explore the wild feminine with a group of women. In the company of others or on your own, you will find many ways to celebrate your feminine radiance. Whatever your history with your body, you can begin now to discover the powerful resources within.

By putting *Wild Feminine* to practice, we learn how to bring strength and vitality to the core. We recognize that skilled body-work will often resolve many of the physical imbalances in the pelvic bowl, providing relief from prolapse, pelvic pain, postpartum muscle imbalances, incontinence, diminished libido, or even just a generalized disconnect, and instead enhance the well-being of our sensual and sexual core and ability to receive pleasure. We can heal psychically from past sexual or pelvic traumas by reclaiming our rightful range. We clear blocks from our core energetic flow and witness a resurgence in our creative capacities. We can revive our feminine and masculine energies to reinvent our jobs, relationships, roles, and other structures that define us in order to be fully expressive and deeply nurtured.

But even more important, we as women can recognize the potential of the pelvic bowl that taps directly into the universal energies, from which all of life is made. By exploring this place where the universal energy meets the female body, we come home to the mystery within us and engage with that mystery to give life to the body, and body to the life.

## My Spirit Daughter

Things always happen to me in the fall. The timing of my miscarriage was no different. The leaves had just a tinge of red when I began to bleed. There were signs of an approaching change, my body's preparation to meet what was coming. Though I had known the same rhythm for many years, I was still unprepared for this event.

Miscarriage is not, as I had always imagined, like an unexpected menstrual period. On the day of my miscarriage, I awoke from a dream that I was bleeding, but my sense of dread did not dissipate upon awakening. The red of my blood confirmed what my body already knew; miscarriage is birth and death simultaneously. Miscarriage is ecstatic connection and unquenchable loss. The uterus dilates and contracts, as in the process of birth. In its wake follows an ancient grief, the grief of grandmothers and women who have lived before, pouring forth from the uterus.

At one point, in the height of uterine contractions, I became drowsy. Surrendering to the path of this unborn soul, I lay down upon the floor. Lying in my place of meditation, near the window framing a large cedar tree, I closed my eyes. Looking back now, I recognize the place of stillness that marks the moment just before a baby emerges from the womb. Breath is suspended and there is infinite quiet, standing at this edge, where once again everything is understood.

Time passed, but I was unaware of its passage until my uterus shuddered. Suddenly, the spirit of my daughter filled the room. I felt her tiny body leave mine, and I reached down to discover her placenta's perfect fit in the palm of my hand.

I wrapped her hint of a body in cloth, not knowing what else to do. With no obvious path set before me, I wandered through the day with her small bundle in my pocket. At sunset, I stood with my son and husband in our backyard. I hesitated, kneeling down at the side of a shallow grave. I did not want to let her go. My hands lifted her out of my pocket and placed her gently against the soft, dark earth. I heard the voice of my son and remembered where I was. My grief rose until the air around me was spinning.

In the days that followed, I embraced the grief in my uterus even though it was easier to ignore it. Working with the female body has shown me that unacknowledged grief never goes away; it simply becomes buried. If a woman denies and buries her bodily grief, she may never walk that region of herself again. Over time she loses access to her own feminine range, sometimes wandering outside of her vital self altogether.

By allowing the grief of my female body to take whatever shape it might, I discovered other forgotten ground. I felt how detached my own uterus had been. I knew myself as a strong woman. Still, I was a stranger in this core place. In the expression of grief and other feelings about losing a baby, I also found grief for not being celebrated as a girl or a woman.

I journeyed into my grief and came upon my first sense of peace. It was peace I had been searching for, and ultimately found, deep within my feminine self. By giving expression to the buried grief of my womanhood, I was exploring the hidden contours of my female body. I was coming home.

Grieving from my womb, I traveled down through layers of stored emotions that had inadvertently blocked access to my root. As I recognized each bit of sadness or loss held in my core, I also realized the heft of the burdens I had been carrying as a woman. In the desire to grieve for the soul of my child, I stepped beyond the boundary of what I had previously allowed myself to feel. Touching the weight of each loss shifted the energy in my core. I was no longer afraid of what I might find. I lifted each stone in my body until I felt the sensation of bare dirt. For the first time I saw a vast inner landscape: the open expanse of my own creative range.

From this root place of connection, I saw my body as an ally. Had I miscarried three years earlier, while pregnant with my first child, I would have tightened every muscle in my pelvis, using my will to silence my womb. Now I was following the lead of my root, trusting the response of my wild feminine.

In the peace of my body, I called to my spirit daughter. Asking how I might remember her, I heard this reply: *Teach women to know the beauty of their bodies and to celebrate the feminine in themselves.*

# ONE

# Beginning Your Journey

*The female body is a sacred space for meeting with spirit.
Women are the weavers of our universe: through their bodies they
take in pure creative essence and then actively create a dynamic form.
Modern women can access this capacity with intention only when
they know how to work with the underlying patterns that shape
their creative range. This chapter examines what is inherently a
mystical creative process within a framework that can be
interacted with and cultivated in daily life, restoring
an intimate relationship to the sacred within.*

*T*he wild feminine is an elusive creature. Like most wild things, she appears when least expected: arising from deep stillness, frequently taking flight just as our awareness responds to her presence. She appears in my work with women the way the wind stirs and blows through an open window. Something clear and deep is restored when women reconnect to this wild place in themselves. In writing this book, my challenge was to define exactly what took place during this process of reconnection, so that women could find their own way there.

At first I did not recognize the wild feminine; my only understanding of the feminine was as a gender construct. But observing her return in the energy and expressions of the women in my midst,

I saw the true feminine nature. When a woman found the wild feminine in her core, she was radiant and wise in her own unique way. All previous notions of what I had called feminine changed, and I was inspired by each encounter with this authentic feminine.

My desire to understand this mysterious feminine essence prompted me to leave my young sons in the care of their father and fly from one coast to another for a women's conference in New York City. Like a biologist in pursuit of a rare animal, I would seek the wild feminine in the places she was likely to appear.

While tending to my children and home in the weeks before I left, I savored the romantic notion of a trip to New York. I would stay with my best girlfriend; in the past five years, she had never seen me without my children. I could satisfy my need for adventure through a solo excursion to the big city.

My New York venture was deliciously appealing from the comfort of my living room, less so in the gritty reality of travel. It was late at night by the time I arrived at my girlfriend's apartment, and my breasts were bulging with milk meant for my youngest son. I retrieved a handheld breast pump from my luggage and attempted to relieve the building pressure. To my dismay, there was no suction in the pump. I then discovered the purpose of a tiny piece of latex left at home. No, that contact lens–sized disk was not just a filter for the milk. It provided suction. Without it, a breast pump just blows air back and forth. I looked in the mirror. At the sight of the harsh light on my milk-laden breasts and my hands pushing and pulling my inept pump in a futile effort to extract a bit of milk, I started to laugh; I even snorted a few times at the absurdity of my situation.

My girlfriend seemed tired. She went to bed, and I was left alone with my engorged melons. "Okay, ladies," I said, hoping that talking to my breasts might encourage their assistance. "I realize you're a little upset. I promise to return you to your baby shortly. Until then, we must make do." I leaned over the sink and began to squeeze. (I would repeat this every four hours in various bathroom stalls at the conference, and then later at the airport, until finally reunited with my breastfeeding son two days later. I hoped my breasts would forgive me.)

Leaving my children and home had made me feel raw, yet my senses also seemed attuned for discovery. The next day I felt alert and prepared for a greater understanding. I left my girlfriend's house early, while New York was still bathed in the gold of morning light. As I found my seat at the conference, the laughter and voices of women were all around me. I was ready to receive the information I was seeking when Marion Woodman began to speak.

Marion, a leading feminine spiritualist and Jungian analyst, has spent a lifetime studying the feminine. If anyone could illuminate the feminine nature, it was she. In general culture, references to women often reflect stereotyped versions of femininity with the term *feminine*. I wondered how Marion would define something or someone as feminine.

Almost as if reading my thoughts, Marion stepped up to the podium, commenting on the beautiful feminine banners, which hung as a backdrop to the stage. After musing about color and texture and their relation to the feminine, Marion looked right at the audience. She said it was difficult to know the true feminine, because *very few people have experienced it.*

These were the words I had traveled across the country to hear. In my own office, one-on-one with women, I was witnessing the return of something I had hardly met before. Marion Woodman confirmed what I'd suspected: notions of femininity surround us, but what we typically define as feminine is not its true form. The actual experience of the feminine is rare, even in the midst of a conference of hundreds of women exploring their femininity. As women, we possess the feminine in our elemental nature. Why then is its presence so elusive?

The truth is that the feminine has never left us—women, and men, have abandoned it. We have forgotten what it means to live by our feminine principles. Living in profound disconnect from the earth, in the frantic pace of life unmoved by our more natural inner rhythms that alternate between expansive creation and restorative retreat, we have precious little time or space to invite the appearance of the feminine. In fact, we will not encounter the feminine until we return to the place we first met her: the female body.

When we restore the internal pelvic landscape—the capacity within our female bodies that supports the presence of the feminine—we witness a return of the feminine to our lives. When we recognize her essence in the root of our bodies, the feminine will no longer be invisible and endangered. Rather than a gender construct that narrows our range of expression, the feminine becomes a living manifestation of our wild selves. Recovering her full range in our feminine core, we receive sustenance from the wild feminine at last.

## The Wild Feminine Landscape

In my work I use words and phrases like *root, feminine terrain,* and *wild feminine ground* or *landscape* to evoke the resonance between the female body and the earth. Words that compare our bodies to the land, where we sow our chosen seeds and learn to grow what will feed us, reveal our truest form as women.

I call the inner range of the female body the wild feminine landscape: a place where we can interact with the energetic and physical patterns that record our relationship to the feminine and define our inherent creative potential. These patterns in the root of our bodies form a filter through which we perceive our creative lives, shaping our experience of womanhood but also giving us the ground to discover our abundance. Presently, our root patterns typically reflect cultural or familial limitations, rather than our authentic nature, and often restrict our creative range. In learning to read the physical and energetic patterns of the pelvic bowl, we can challenge these restrictions and reacquaint ourselves with our full feminine landscape.

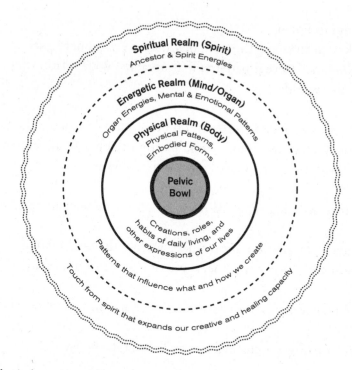

Physical tension and energetic blocks in the pelvic bowl limit core vitality and energy flow. Conversely, physical alignment and balanced energy patterns create robust health and the potential for greater flow and energy resources into our bodies and lives.

We live in our bodies. We have thoughts and identities, relationship patterns and emotional patterns. We tend to think of the patterns in our bodies and the patterns of our lives as permanent forms, but each—from our deepest cells to the vastness of our creative capacity—is a dynamic expression that can evolve and change, and respond to the environment that surrounds it. By exploring the body, mind, and spirit aspects of our female forms, we encounter both the possible limitations that may restrict our femininity as well as the source for our inspired expression. Rather than a solid structure, we discover the vibrant nature that exists in and around us.

## Changing Form

The key to changing the form that shapes your inner landscape is to examine the internal patterns that organize your relationship with the outer world:

1. Proprioceptive maps (based on perception of space and position arising from sense stimuli within the body) are patterns formed from the internal sense of body awareness.

2. Kinesthetic maps record information for movement patterns.

3. Layers of tension or softness within the body often give meaning to sensory information or emotional information.

4. Mental constructs give form to what is expected or possible.

5. Inner pathways channel energy flow in the body.

Together, these patterns interact to inform your daily movements, habits, ways of being, and potential for engaging with each experience. Working with and realigning these patterns for body awareness, movement, tension, mental habits, and energy flow can change how you embody—or literally inhabit your body—and utilize your creative energy. Though we have these patterns and layers throughout the body, we will focus on the pelvic bowl and the root patterns that define creative flow.

To reconnect with the root of your body and begin the process of working with your own form, you must first encounter the energy of long-held, often unconscious, emotions and mental attitudes (patterns) preventing you from cherishing your womanhood and accessing your core radiance. As you meditate on your pelvic bowl and identify the history held in your core, you will learn what feminine aspects you have come to value or disregard for yourself. You will begin to recognize how patterns you carry can diminish your own abundance or cause you to live outside of your center. You may not know the stories of your ancestors, nor how those stories have formed the range of your feminine self, but you can look to the energy in your pelvic bowl and discover the gifts and challenges of your heritage and how they affect your energy flow. By clearing energetic obstacles from your core or studying your root energy patterns, you can reshape inherited patterns associated with feminine roles or the use of your creative energies, and experience delightful new ways of physically, energetically, and spiritually embodying your feminine form.

## Feminine and Masculine Energy

Most of the information in this book relates to the feminine. Of course, every person has both feminine and masculine energy, designed to complement one another. The feminine is the in-breath, the internal tide of intuition and inspiration that shapes and influences the out-breath, or masculine form. When balanced, the feminine and masculine result in creative abundance, and the forms that arise from this balance are both productive and sustainable.

Masculine energy, when balanced by the feminine, is robust and playful, able to create with beauty and pleasure in its formations. However, we are presently experiencing a profound division between masculine and feminine that is evident in our bodies and lives. The absence of the feminine and the domination of a distorted masculine is both destructive and unsustainable, manifesting many structures that are harmful to the earth and our very existence. As we restore our connection to the feminine, we will witness the rise of a vibrant masculine. (I explore the masculine and feminine divide, as well as the potential for healing, in chapter 4.)

Working with the root of our bodies, we can realign and redefine these physical and energetic patterns that otherwise restrict the energy flow in our bodies and lives. Clearing stagnant energy and emotional burdens from the pelvic bowl, we have more creative energy to use as we desire. Changing our core patterns, we clarify the filter through which we experience our womanhood and transform the way that we receive energy or give life to our creations.

In the womb, our bodies take shape: spirit first becomes body. If we understand this potential in the root, of bringing spirit into form, we recognize the energy of the spiritual realm as essential for infusing our lives with joy and building our creative dreams. We perceive life as greater than the situations we encounter and allow the energy of spirit to flow through the core of our beings, bringing vitality and inspiration to each moment. Our embodied forms, whether as physical bodies, creative designs, partnerships, or the structures we build within our lives, become alive, responsive, radiant—in other words, wild—an outer expression of our full and finest creative selves.

## Women's Stories: Realizing the Feminine for Herself

Jill was referred to me by a friend who had experienced the profound impact of reconnecting with her pelvic space, so Jill wanted to discover what blocked her own pelvic connection. In learning about her pelvic imbalances, Jill noticed her tendency to distance herself from anything that she thought of as feminine.

She found it difficult to bring awareness to her pelvic space. She was hardly present in this part of her body. Jill noted that in her family, the men were respected and the women were overlooked, and she felt she had rejected her femininity in response to the limitations she associated with being female. As a young girl, she had identified herself as a tomboy. Later, when she began to menstruate, she felt embarrassed and ashamed by this monthly reminder of her femininity. Rather than welcoming the arrival of her womanhood, Jill rejected her period as a sign of weakness.

Rejecting her femininity ultimately limited Jill's own expression of the feminine. Avoiding feminine associations prevented her from accessing the creativity, vitality, and passion that comes from a strong feminine connection.

Jill and I began our work together by discussing the wisdom of her womb cycles. Alternately holding or releasing the menstrual lining, the uterus provides direction for a woman, signaling when to move boldly into the world or, alternately, when to rest. The idea of synchronizing her outer movements with the natural rhythms of her body inspired her, encouraging her to shed her previous sense of shame.

As we worked with her body, Jill found it difficult to maintain mental focus on her vagina. This disconnection expressed itself physically as well: she was aware of sensation in some areas of her vaginal muscles, yet in others, she felt numb. I encouraged her to breathe and take notice of each region in her pelvic bowl. As I pressed my finger along each point of her internal pelvic rim, Jill could feel the bowl formed by the bones of her pelvis. Repeatedly directing her awareness back to her root body sensations, Jill also noticed an immense sadness inside herself.

By simply observing her sadness, and breathing toward her pelvic space, Jill found that her feelings had a wave-like quality. A wave of sadness would rise, increase in intensity, then soften and eventually dissipate. In the place where she felt the sadness, Jill became aware of a basic, almost primal need for touch and connection. She was surprised by the force and clarity of the desires arising from her feminine core. In the root of her body, Jill found a fierce determination.

Discovering an unwavering strength in her female body challenged Jill's notion of femininity as weak. Paying attention to her root on a daily basis, Jill began to consciously reevaluate her perceptions of the feminine. Each time she brought awareness to her pelvic bowl, she encountered the same sense of clarity and direction. Over time, Jill reframed her own femininity; rather than perceiving it as a weakness, she began to relate and respond to her feminine nature, reawakening to this resource within her female body.

Jill changed her relationship with her body, and she observed a profound change in the quality of her sexual intimacy. Prior to our work, Jill typically felt distant from her partner after having sex. Unsatisfied by their lovemaking, she tried meeting her needs by talking about her frustrations. But her partner felt criticized and Jill felt unheard, leaving the situation continually unresolved.

As Jill became attuned to her root, she became more aware of her body during lovemaking. She was aware of a wider range of sensations and emotions, making the overall experience of sex more physical and spontaneous. By focusing on her pelvic bowl, Jill was more aroused by her partner's masculine presence. Her partner responded with his body to the deeper connection she had with her own body, and they were both more nourished by their sexual exchange.

Whether following the guidance from her pelvic bowl or discovering a relationship with the feminine in her core, Jill had found a multitude of different ways to receive and then create with her own feminine energy.

## Ecology of Woman

Ecology refers to the series of interrelated relationships made between a specific organism and its outer world. As an undergraduate, I studied ecology and was fascinated by the interplay of relationships within each environment. Every living thing has an ecology, or various ways of communicating and connecting with its surroundings. Women too have their own ecology: the rhythms of our natural inner cycles that serve to guide us in our interactions with the outer world. This interaction between our female bodies and our feminine landscapes is where we cultivate and transform our creations. When we change the patterns in the pelvic bowl and utilize the energy of our organs with consciousness, we also change the energy we draw from our environment and the capacity for manifesting our creations.

## The Womb Cycle

The primary ecological exchange in the female body occurs through the womb cycle. Each organ of the pelvic space plays its part in the womb cycle in a series of smaller, interconnected cycles that I have named cycle of transformation, cycle of creation, and cycle of regeneration.

*Note: Even if a woman has had a hysterectomy or one of her ovaries removed, she can cultivate her organ energies. The organ's original place in her body still functions as the energy center associated with that particular organ. In the section below, I also describe the womb cycle as if a woman is still menstruating to illustrate the rhythmic nature of the female body. Regardless of her reproductive status, or even if she has entered menopause, the energy of the female body continues to move in outward expansion and restorative retreat in alignment with the full and new moons or personal creative and life cycles. I encourage all women to learn their own internal rhythms by paying attention to the physical and energetic changes in their bodies.*

The uterus contains the cycle of transformation. Like the ocean tide moving in and out with the magnetic pull of the moon, the uterus has its own blood tide. The uterine lining thickens, swells, and then thins in a rhythmic pattern. In my own body, and working with women, I have noticed that during the buildup of the menstrual lining, the uterus energetically and physically gestates a woman's creations, giving her more energy for her desired projects. When the uterus sheds its lining, a woman's body releases the energy she no longer needs and invites her to rest and refocus before beginning another creative cycle. I associate the womb cycle with transformation because it is most closely related to birth and death and the intimate workings of the creative process. We have birth and death cycles—where new energy enters and old energy is released—in every season of our lives.

The ovaries maintain the cycle of creation, each alternately releasing an egg and sending it to the womb. I relate the ovarian cycle to creation because the ovaries contain all of a woman's potential creative seeds. Observing ovarian energy patterns in my clients, I have found that the left ovary draws energy from the feminine aspect of the body. Receiving energy inward, in the receptive manner of the feminine, the left ovary can be a source of inspiration and replenishment for a woman's creative cycle. The right ovary, on the other hand, draws energetically from the masculine aspect of the body. Putting energy outward, in the projective manner of the masculine, the right ovary gives form and expression to a woman's creations. Together, the ovaries balance these complementary energies in the female body and pelvic bowl. We live in a more balanced way, with an abundance of both personal inspiration and vibrant expression, when we access the full potential of our feminine and masculine energies.

As the gatekeeper, the vagina regulates the cycle of regeneration. I associate the vagina with regeneration because at various times during the womb cycle, the vagina is open to receive or release as necessary to revitalize the female body. When a woman is fertile and open to receive new inspiration, the muscles of the vagina become softer and there is an increase in lubrication to receive the sexual energy of her partner. The muscles also soften to release her uterine lining during menstruation when her body sheds what is no longer needed. Conversely, the vagina becomes drier and vaginal muscles more engaged when a woman's body is integrating what was received or building the uterine lining. With a solid connection to the vagina, a woman is more in touch with her own sensual nature and ability to receive pleasure, even in everyday life.

The organ cycles of the female pelvis are synergistic, each working together to support, inspire, and transform a woman's creative potential. These are physical cycles: the rhythms of ovarian eggs, uterine blood, vaginal lubrication or changes in pelvic muscle tone, as well as pregnancy and childbirth. But more subtly and powerfully, these cycles involve the flow of energy, the essential life force. Regardless of her stage in life, a woman interacts with this life force energy in her pelvic bowl.

When women cultivate the energy of the womb through breath and conscious awareness of the fertility or inner creative cycle, they witness physical changes. My clients have reported shifts in the length or timing of their periods, the color of menstrual blood, physical sensations, pelvic tone, vaginal lubrication, and uterine fluids. They also report having more access to their intuitive wisdom and clarity in using their creative energy. When women pay attention to female ecology, they also relate differently to their bodies. They describe enhanced feelings of connection, pride, and awe for the amazing female body. This, in turn, impacts the way a woman relates to her environment. Every time I hear a woman speak with renewed respect for her root, I have hope for the future of girls, boys, and partners associated with these women who know how to celebrate the female form.

## Art, Ritual, and the Flow of Pelvic Energy

In Western culture and medicine, the word *energy* connotes something New Age but not tangible or real. Yet many cultures and ancient medical practices recognize energy as the restorative life force that circulates throughout the body to enliven the cells and facilitate good health. In yoga and Ayurvedic medicine, this energy is known as prana. In Oriental medicine, it is referred to as *chi*.

The quality of energy flow in the female pelvis, including the flow of each ovary, the uterus, and the vagina, impacts a woman's overall vibrancy. Like nutrients drawn from the soil that are essential for a plant's growth, the flow of pelvic energy through a woman's root determines the vitality of her womanhood. The root of her body contains a woman's creative energy system, which includes both the first and second chakras (energy centers that regulate core identity and creative expression) and the energy of her pelvic bowl and female organs. When a woman understands how to utilize this system, she can change or cultivate the energy she holds in her center.

When energy is blocked in a woman's root, either by physical tension, emotional burden, past trauma, or long-term patterns of core energy imbalance, it inhibits the energy flow in her life. By learning how to evaluate her pelvic energy, a woman can identify these blocks to her vitality. Accessing her uterine and ovarian energies with the exercises provided in this book, she can clear the energy of her pelvic bowl and clarify her everyday use of energy. Freeing her core energy from emotional burdens or even family lineage patterns that limit her creative flow, she discovers more creative energy for her own life.

Initially, in my work to restore balance in a woman's pelvic bowl, I would do an extensive internal massage to release the pelvic tension in her core muscles. As my awareness for the power of energy movement in the body increased, I began to have women direct their breath and internal focus to the area I was massaging. This focused more energy on the region and I found that the muscle tension dissolved almost immediately. In holistic medicine practices, the primary blockages in the body are thought to be energetic in nature; these energy obstructions are believed to cause physical symptoms. Although my practice of women's health is based in physical medicine, I have found that there is much less structural work to be done in the pelvis when a woman addresses her root energy patterns.

Every woman possesses internal awareness of her body. If you close your eyes, you still know where your arm is positioned in space because you have that internal awareness (proprioception) of your arm. Energy movement in the body responds to internal awareness and focused breathing; by visualizing a certain region of your body and directing your breath there, you can cultivate your own energy. It is easier to be more aware of, and able to focus on, the parts of the body that are frequently moved or used, like hands and feet.

Since the pelvic bowl does not receive regular attention, most women lack a sense of internal awareness about this part of their body except with sexual intercourse or upon giving birth. From day to day, they do not give the pelvic bowl much thought. Still, by working with breath and visualization, focused meditation on the pelvic bowl, or hands-on vaginal massage, you can become more aware of and can even affect the energy of your core—bringing more creative flow into your daily life.

### Exercise: Visualizing the Pelvic Bowl

1. Bring your awareness to your pelvic bowl. See if you can find the edges of this bowl. Even if you aren't sure of your exact physical anatomy, picture your bowl in your mind's eye and walk around the outer edges, moving your awareness around your bowl in a circle. Notice the shape and other qualities of your bowl. Is it round and even on all sides?

2. The inner fibers and energy of the pelvic bowl are reminiscent of a bird's nest. Notice if any part of the bowl feels pushed in,

dent-like, or diffuse so that the edge is difficult to perceive. These may be areas where you have lost touch with this inner feminine range: the intuitive and creative expanse of your feminine expression.

3. Bring your breath to any area that is not soft or rounded and see what changes. Imagine smoothing the energy of your pelvic bowl just as a bird smoothes and shapes its nest.

4. When the process feels complete, finish by giving thanks for your pelvic bowl, the core of your feminine ground.

## The Female Body: Your Own Creative Landscape

The female body is designed to be creative. Actively cultivating your personal creative expression is essential for revitalizing your creative energy. Creating from your center moves the energy of your core. Though we tend to label certain people as artists, any woman who cherishes her creative essence will find herself making art: children, gardens, meals, altars, new ways of living, and other vibrant creations. A woman who accesses her creativity as an artist, teacher, or visionary may experience the joy of her root when working on a specific creation. However, if she only uses her creativity in one area, her energy becomes compartmentalized. Your creative essence is a tremendous resource; it is meant to flow as a unifying force that weaves together the total expression of your feminine potential.

The creative process is designed to be sustainable, with abundant energy both for you and your heartfelt creations. The natural rhythm of the womb offers guidance for how and when to create in a manner that replenishes the energy in your body. Attuning yourself to the cyclical movement of your womb in planning your creations, you will find yourself following a creative wave and feeling restored, rather than depleted, as you travel with each creative cycle.

There are many ways to discover your internal flow of pelvic energy and to increase your ability to access this creative potential of your root. Using physical and energetic pelvic care tools to restore the whole energy movement in the pelvic bowl expands your creative capacity. Developing a personal relationship with the feminine allows you to take in more chi (energy) to create with. Perhaps the most powerful way you can increase pelvic energy flow is to create while following your joy, providing a place for your feminine spirit to play.

When creating in a manner that brings you joy, your body draws energy *in* (feminine movement) from the environment and puts it *out* (masculine movement) in a particular form. You may be writing, painting, mothering, dancing, cooking, decorating, or otherwise using your creative essence in a playful rather than solely productive manner; when doing so, energy moves through your pelvis. You can be productive in your joy as well, for example, by clearing a room to enhance the positive energy flow (known as improving the feng shui, a process of aligning a room) or working on a project that inspires you, but the key is sensing the movement of energy in your center. If you feel energized in the process, then energy is flowing rather than simply becoming depleted. As energy flows in the pelvic bowl, it replenishes the energy of the female body and gives expression to the feminine spirit. This type of creative play will lead you to your best creations, producing what truly matters to you and in a seasonal manner.

As you recover the wisdom of your inherent creative cycles and learn how your body may direct you toward particular creative seeds and periods of active creation or quiet restoration, you may discover blocks to your creative process. For example, some women initiate creative projects but have difficulty sustaining them. Others can initiate and sustain a project but are challenged by bringing it to completion. Some women pursue an abundance of inspirations without recognizing their own internal creative direction. Others are unable to tap into their own creative fire and rely on outside inspiration or attempt to make the fire of others their own.

Creative blocks can be felt in the root as physical or emotional tension, and are typically the result of blockages in the female energy system. Working with these blocks will restore the full energetic range of each organ in the creative cycle. When encountering a creative block, either as tension in the pelvic bowl, stagnant energy, or frustration with your creative direction, you can recognize the block's purpose: paying attention to a creative block (rather than simply trying to be rid of it) often teaches you how to re-access a particular energy flow in your body or a part of your creative range. Working with the blocks to align your core energy is like bringing the process of feng shui to the pelvic bowl. Meeting obstacles in this manner makes them more manageable, even a source of inspiration.

Every woman is inherently creative, but most creative energy is used in a limited way, within specific circumstances or certain roles. When you understand how to engage your creative energy and increase its flow in your body—and *all* areas of your life—you find your real potential for creation and transformation.

### *Exercise: Spontaneous Creation*

Try this exercise any time you want to stir the creative energy in your bowl.

1. Bring awareness down to your root. Place your hand over your pelvis and try to sense how it feels just beneath your hand. Is this area warm or cold, tight or open, quiet or active? Notice the quality of energy here. Some women feel particular sensations (prickly, hot, or soft) when sensing energy, while others see colors or light.

2. After reflecting for a moment on the energy in your core, select a medium for spontaneous expression. For five minutes, freewrite, color, dance, sing, play, or move your creative energy in whatever way appeals to you. Let yourself follow the movement arising from your center.

3. After five minutes of creation, return your attention back to your body. Again notice the quality of energy or sensations in your pelvic bowl. What has changed? What has happened with your energy?

## The Importance of Ritual and Creative Intention

Ritual is a creative movement with a specific intention. It is an invitation to the presence of the divine, using the power of symbols to establish connections with the members of a woman's community, the sacred, or something larger than yourself. Ritual, with certain patterns or objects that are involved in its structure, is a form that holds and moves energy. When repeated, a ritual has more physical and energetic structure, more power to assist the movement and transformation of energy. This book offers a sampling of rituals, simple actions that honor the feminine and cultivate divine energy in a woman's body. Every woman has the ability to celebrate the sacred feminine in herself. In celebration, she transforms what is held in the center of her being.

Like art, ritual moves energy and is a vital component for restoring the energy flow in the pelvic bowl. When you do a ritual or create sacred space in your feminine realm, you invite the presence of spirit into your creative work and daily life. The act of ritualizing gives form to the intangible aspects of grieving a loss or healing a wound of the spirit, moving the energies these wounds contain, and making more room for the raw material of creation. As you make your own rituals and return to them over time, they serve you as a source of comfort and deepen their potential for healing or celebrating in your life.

One of my favorite rituals is one that I can do even in the midst of my busy household. It clears the energy of my pelvic bowl and plants my creative intentions. A creative intention may represent something that I am working on that day, or it may be part of a more elaborate creative design; either way, I honor myself when I recognize the power and divine potential of planting intentions directly in my core.

### Exercise: Clearing the Pelvic Bowl and Planting Your Creative Intentions

1. Close your eyes and focus on your pelvic bowl. Take a moment to notice the quality of energy in this root place.

2. Now begin to walk the edges of your bowl, starting in front and moving to the right. As you go, use your breath and imagine sweeping your arms to clear the energy in the bowl. Give your body permission to clear anything that is no longer needed, any energy blocking your access to spirit or your own beauty, and visualize this excess energy as light or water that moves down, through your root, into the ground.

3. When you have finished walking a complete circle, sweeping out your whole bowl, go to the center of your bowl. Here, in your center, is the energy of your uterus. Sitting in your center, ask yourself, "What is my greatest creative dream?" See what comes to you, whether as words, images, or simply an invitation for new energy. Then ask, "What will nourish the seeds of my dream?" Again, see what comes. Plant what you have learned as intentions in your core.

4. Take one more walk around this newly planted ground and ask for only helpful energies, drawing from the realm of

spirit, to come and surround you. Bring this visualization to a close and give thanks for your pelvic bowl, the root for all your creations.

## How to Begin

Reclaiming the wild feminine means tending to your own feminine nature. It involves contemplating what has shaped your feminine identity and deciding which core patterns serve your well-being and which are in need of a new form. The core physical and energetic patterns held in your pelvic bowl channel the flow of your creative energy, affecting your vitality and what you are able to create. However, these core patterns can be changed once you understand how they define your creative range. To begin exploring this inner wild feminine landscape and learning how it shapes your outer world, start with a specific realm of the feminine that draws your attention.

Perhaps you may choose to begin by focusing on the physical aspect of your feminine core. Connect with the physical layers in your pelvic bowl through massage, exercise, or conscious care. Or you can work with the energy layers—by clearing energy blocks and enabling flow—to enhance your pelvic vitality. The physical layers are the most dense and therefore respond to a more direct approach, such as touch. The energetic layers are less dense and respond to lighter contact, such as focused breath and visualization exercises. Paying attention to your sensations and your internal sense will encourage your awareness for the connection between the physical and energetic layers. When changing core patterns, it is helpful to work on both the physical and energetic layers—and to understand the relationship between them—to achieve more profound and lasting results.

As you reflect on the wild feminine and the patterns within your body, explore the ways that you currently experience your

femininity. Do you follow the inherent rhythms of your female
body? Is there a spiritual expression of the feminine that you
desire? What was it like to be a woman in your family? How do
you express your femininity? Where is your femininity blocked or
inaccessible? When have you felt restricted by definitions of femininity? By attuning yourself to various regions of the feminine, and
the expression of the feminine in body and energy flow, you can
consciously cultivate feminine energy and restore your full, wild
feminine range.

### Examples of Cultivating Your Wild Feminine Landscape

1. Physical patterns: Reduce tension and increase dynamic
   engagement in the core through vaginal massage, self-care,
   exercise, awareness of body sensations, daily habits that support core health, a practice of mindfulness, and reduction
   of stress.

2. Energetic patterns: Strengthen and clarify your energy with
   breathing/visualization exercises, cultivating pelvic organ
   energies, accessing a full range of organ energies, following
   inherent creative cycles, moving stagnant emotional energies,
   clearing negative energies from the core, and filling it with
   positive, loving energies.

3. Linking physical form with energy flow: Observe the
   physical and energetic balance in the core and how it effects
   your daily creative flow (the movement of energy that you
   use to create your life); reinforce areas of ease and heal parts
   of your creative and sensual expression that have stagnated;
   change the structure of roles, routines, ways of being, or any
   limiting forms to better express your dynamic nature; make
   clear agreements that reflect your value and true desires;

incorporate ritual, a relationship with wild places and the sacred, a bodily experience of the feminine, and a connection to lineage to enrich your energy potential.

## Run Your Creative Energy with Intention

As women, we run energy through our bodies and into our lives. This way of nurturing and creating, by channeling the vibrant energy of the universe through the body, is uniquely female and belongs to each woman. Though we actively run our creative energy—building our lives; tending to partners, children, careers; or all of the above—we often do this unconsciously, without noticing what is happening in the root. This energy can be protective, healing, and revitalizing for us, but only when used with intention.

To be intentional about the flow of creative energy means examining how you have learned to use your creative essence. Expending this energy to the point of exhaustion, giving more than you are taking in, or tying the use of your energy to your value or a sense of obligation are all unsustainable patterns that will deplete your life force. Women often use their creative life force because they want to be *good*, having internalized cultural messages that encourage them to put the needs of others before their own. We do true good when we are more discerning in the use of our creative capacity.

Before accessing your creative energy for any endeavor, sense how you really feel about the project or request. If you feel pressured, ask yourself why. If you feel bad about saying no, again ask yourself why. The only reason to say yes is when you feel a rising tide of energy in your center. In this way, your body is connecting you to a deeper current that will feed you, even as you give of yourself. To be able to run your creative energy with intention, you must be present in your pelvic bowl and heal any patterns that connect your creative energy to a need for value or validation. When you are clear on your inherent value, you understand that your creative energy is a precious resource to cultivate with care and to invest with joy.

## Collect Your Feminine Resources

Acknowledge your feminine resources as essential support for recovering your wild femininity. These include the personal talents and capabilities that you already have as well as those you may potentially access in the various feminine realms. For example, using the physical strength of your pelvic muscles builds core stability in your body. Clearing the energy of the pelvic bowl provides clarity, enhances capacity for those creations that are truly inspiring, and makes room for the vast resources of spirit. Embracing your full emotional spectrum releases emotional burdens and enriches your depth of feeling for each experience of womanhood. Using your cycle of fertility naturally replenishes the energy you bring to creative projects.

Collecting your feminine resources can also mean honoring the gifts you receive in the context of female community. By acknowledging the wisdom of other women, you find your own place of contribution while also learning additional skills. Perhaps you bring laughter and lightness to an occasion, while another woman offers a sense of reflection. One mother teaches self-expression through physical play; another helps her child find his voice in storytelling. One woman gathers people together, while another paints in her studio. Each woman contributes in her own way, engaging the environment uniquely: together they fill the needs of the community.

Utilize the support available in a community of women and share the power. Look to the women within your community for the projects and creative works that inspire your own creations, and honor those whose work paves the way. Follow your joy to classes, professional networking groups, or other events that allow you to connect with vibrant women. Create your own circles by gathering on the full moon to share what each of you is presently creating, inviting women to participate in rituals together, making a shared dinner and reflecting on a theme regarding the feminine, having a creative night for women to work on projects while enjoying female company. Meeting with other women is powerful way to revitalize your own creative energy.

As you come to know your wild feminine, you will identify your natural resources as well as those you would like to develop. Resources also include practitioners offering skilled guidance for navigating difficult regions of your healing path, so seek assistance from your community of healthcare and spiritual providers to further address your needs. Call upon spirit, ancestors, and the spirits of the land with ritual and prayer. You are not alone on this journey, and it is wise to have support for processing your feelings, moving the energies, and creating new patterns as you cultivate your wild feminine range.

Reflections on collecting your feminine resources include:

What are your natural resources?
What resources would you like to gather for healing?
What resources are available in your community of women?
What personal resources have you yet to access?

In working with women, I have seen that healing the pelvic patterns of imbalance and disconnection also links each woman to universal aspects of womanhood. For example, one woman may be recovering from miscarriage, while another is learning how to cherish herself: both may work through issues of shame held in the body to restore a sense of wholeness in their femininity. One of my motivations for writing this book was to offer a perspective that allows women to understand their personal experiences within a greater community context.

When a woman accesses her own root wisdom, she joins this universal female community. Your ecology, the link between your body and your outer world, is your connection with other women. What seems unbearable in isolation may become tolerable with the support of shared experiences. It is my intention that the women's stories in this book remind you that you are not alone. May the words of these stories bring hope and guidance in healing your feminine wounds and unfolding your feminine potential.

This personal journey is the basis for a global transformation: each of us making our way back to ourselves, forging the tools that enable our passage. Awakening to the most feminine part of our female bodies, we are beginning to heal and nurture our wild femininity. Restoring a bodily connection to the feminine, we are opening the channel for spirit and radiant energy to flow more readily into our lives. Together, we are planting the seeds that will grow to nourish the soul of the wild feminine in our culture at large.

## A Little Effort Goes a Long Way

If the thought of redefining your feminine identity, acknowledging your feminine wounds, or rebuilding the structure of your pelvic bowl and creative energy flow seems a bit overwhelming, remember that a little effort goes a long way. Just as your self-concept as a woman affects many realms of your life, each step you make in relating to and cherishing your femininity will have multiple positive impacts. Some of these impacts you may notice, such as feeling more at ease in your body or in your ability to express yourself. Other changes may be less noticeable, yet equally powerful. For example, you may start to prioritize your creativity or be more conscious of your language in ways that have great influence over time.

Working with the wild feminine is like tending a piece of land; work done day by day in a sustainable way builds upon itself and transforms the landscape. The following self-care list from one of my clients is a beautiful example of simple and practical ways to address feminine needs:

**My self-care:**
- Massaging tender spots in pelvic muscles
- Breathing to release pelvic holding
- Acknowledging anger, pain, and resentment associated with motherhood
- Acknowledging grief at the loss of my son's infancy
- Thanking my body for my baby and for its hard work

**Healing actions:**
- Lit candles symbolizing grandmothers who passed away and acknowledged their spirits
- Spoke with fourteen-month-old son about grandmothers and lineage
- Wrote in journal

**Want to focus further on:**
- Reconciling the anger at my body regarding my challenging pregnancy
- Finding ways to process and move my anger
- Checking in and talking with my uterus on a regular basis

The tools for addressing your feminine needs are available right here in your own pelvic bowl. Your female body contains your greatest creative resources: they belong to you when you access this potential in your root.

The experiences that lead us as women to psychically and spiritually disconnect from the roots of our bodies (and the full capacity of our creative range) vary, but one fundamental issue maintains this separation: the spirit naturally moves away from places that are dishonored. The female body is still often a source of shame rather than a place of celebrated, sacred space. The feminine nature is widely perceived as unnecessary or even a weakness. We will not inhabit our dishonored regions; hence, we become blocked in the root, cut off from our source of feminine power.

As women, we belong in a sacred space. Our female bodies are sacred, we carry the future for our daughters and sons, and we have the potential to change the limiting patterns from the generations that went before us. The creative life force moves through us. When we remember that this movement is sacred, we remember the wild in ourselves—this raw and blessed spirit that is uniquely feminine—and in doing so find our expression, our own celebration of life.

*May you discover your infinite creative potential.*

# TWO

# Exploring Your Feminine Ground

*The female body deserves more care; in order to receive more care,
women must understand the language of the body. This chapter
teaches how to read the physical patterns held in the pelvic muscles
and alleviate tension patterns that inhibit energy flow.
Modern women are carrying chronic tension in the pelvis that
interferes with physical and energetic flow in the whole female body.
By learning to pay attention to her own root patterns, a woman can
enhance the flow in her core. Though vaginal self-massage may
be intimidating, all women benefit from learning this and other
tools that encourage them to take true care of their bodies.*

want to share what I have learned from the female body. First, a
woman's body always tells the truth for her. When a woman is
angry, for example, the muscles around her vagina are hot to the
touch. In spring, or when her belly is full with baby, the energy of
her pelvic bowl is bright with new potential. If a woman is lonely
and afraid, the root will convey what is required for her to let down
her guard. Alternately, when a woman is resting and eating well, her
root will be different than when she is under stress.

Know this about the female body: spirit inhabits its sacred
ground. I sat once with my hand on the belly of a woman who
had lost her baby in childbirth. In the lonely days that followed,
she found her body a continual reminder of her daughter's

passing. A deeply spiritual woman, she struggled to feel her daughter's spirit.

I expected only to sit with this woman in the silence of her grief, my hand offering whatever comfort might counter the coldness in her womb. We sat together, two women, my hand on her belly and quiet between us. Suddenly the room became warm. My eyes were closed, but I opened them to see who was standing at my side. I saw no one, yet there was a tremendous presence and warmth beside my body.

My hand was still resting on the woman's belly, and I had the distinct sensation of another hand settling on top of mine. My hand and shoulder felt warm. The warmth spread through my body to her belly, and filled the entire room. We sat, held together by an exquisite tenderness and the truth that a sacred doorway lies in every woman's womb.

When this woman opened her eyes, they were wet with tears. She had seen her baby, just above her body, as we worked. She said that her baby was reaching down to touch her belly. I had been touched as well. My hand and shoulder radiated a gentle heat for the rest of the day. My heart still carries the imprint of this mother and daughter reaching across the doorway to hold and behold each other, a gift of boundless love from spirit.

Connecting with the female body is usually more subtle—but no less profound. We all have this access to spirit in our wombs, for touching the losses in the root of our bodies opens us to spirit. The deepest losses offer the widest openings for us to receive the miracles in our midst, and the more open we are to receive, the more spirit can send to us. But this alignment with spirit requires a willingness to look within and see what is there.

## Take Care of Your Root

The state of her body and the way a woman has learned to inhabit her physical form are revealed by the way she moves in the world.

An erect and open posture indicates comfort with meeting others. A flexed posture shows a preference for the internal realm. Postures can arise from basic personality, but they are also shaped by individual experience. On a more subtle level, postures are formed by tension patterns in the muscles and connective tissue of the body. These patterns encode thousands of encounters and continually influence a woman's interactions and ways of being. The patterns held in the root not only affect the health of a woman's core, they often reflect her experience of being female.

Bodyworkers (physical therapists, chiropractors, and osteopaths) learn how to read and interpret physical patterns. As a physical therapist, I assess which patterns are giving support to the body and enhance the physical structure, and which are inhibiting vitality and require adjustment. The first task for a woman exploring her feminine ground is to learn the tension patterns of her own root.

The root of the female body is the physical ground where a woman can begin to understand her own relationship with the wild feminine. If she brings her attention to the physical structure of her pelvic bowl defined by muscle and bone, she will learn the patterns of her root and discover the ways that her body has internalized or embodied her femininity. Where she feels free to express herself and where she feels more restricted—the range of her wild feminine—is echoed in her core tension patterns. Mapping these patterns and visualizing the anatomy of her pelvic bowl, a woman may discover what physical and energetic patterns define her creative space.

The patterns of the root, the shape of a woman's wild feminine range, can be changed and expanded. Using tools such as vaginal massage, she restores vitality to the root muscles (her pelvic floor), the strongest and most integral muscles supporting the female body. By working with her root, a woman's awareness for more subtle sensations is refined. She will begin to feel the warmth of her own creative energy and recognize how she holds this energy in her pelvic bowl. She will find the connection between the state of her root and her creative capacity. Cultivating and protecting her creative center, she will establish real sustenance in her core.

Caring for the root of her body is a way for a woman to begin speaking with her divine feminine voice. Of course, this dialogue will also remind her of any pain associated with her womanhood, but by acknowledging the layers of wounds and gifts held in her core, a woman opens a path of healing for her spirit. Only by sorting through what she carries does she claim this feminine territory as her own. Newly discovered pain or blockages become landmarks on the pelvic map; a woman's awareness of these blocks allows for their restoration.

When we take care of our bodies at the root, we come to know and love this feminine place in ourselves. By honoring ourselves here, in the center, we give more room for our wild feminine to roam. Reflections on taking care of your root include:

Where do you feel free or blocked in your expression?
How does this reflect your relationship with your body?
Where would you like more capacity for expression or energy flow in your body?

## Learning to Care for the Female Body

Sonya was a client without specific pelvic concerns, but she came for pelvic work because of past experiences integrating mind and body healing practices. She found that whenever she healed something for herself in both mind and body, the result was more profound. With a college degree in women's studies, Sonya was socially empowered by her study of women's issues and felt that learning about pelvic care would empower her in another way.

By taking care of her root, Sonya would learn about the connection between the physical realm of her female body and other aspects of her femininity, such as her emotional state and pelvic energy. While working with women in the pelvic space, I have noticed particular patterns of pelvic tension often correlating with women's experiences in the outer world. These connections between various realms of the feminine are particularly visible in the pelvic map, a tool I teach clients to use as part of their self-care.

When I began working as a physical therapist in women's health, my attention was focused entirely on the pelvic muscles. But in providing hands-on care to the female body, I gained a deeper perspective on how the state of the pelvic bowl affects each woman's feminine experience. Addressing every pelvic symptom, area of tension, or imbalance may assist a woman in reclaiming the potential of her body and cultivating her true feminine nature. For example, balancing the pelvic energy may require that a woman expand her self-expression, grieve a past wound, or restore a lost creative pursuit. In this way, pelvic imbalances offer guidance for rediscovering the wider range of the wild feminine landscape.

## A Pelvic Care Session

I began my work with Sonya, as I have learned to do with all my clients, by orienting her to the female pelvis. First, we talked about the bowl shape of the pelvic bones as well as the pelvic floor— the muscles at the base, quite literally the floor of the pelvic bowl. I described the position of the uterus as the deep center of the pelvic bowl and explained how the other structures often orient around the uterus. The bladder is slightly lower and in front of the uterus, the rectum is behind, and the ovaries are slightly up and to either side. Sonya was curious about the information I was sharing, never having considered this part of her body in such detail.

I described to Sonya the pelvic session and self-care techniques she would be learning. A pelvic care session differs from an annual pelvic exam in several ways. Rather than using a speculum, one finger is placed into the vagina to assess the pelvic muscles. Because the vagina is in the center of the pelvic floor muscles, it provides a perfect access point for evaluating pelvic muscular health.

Though initially many women are hesitant to have a provider touch them in such a private place, and perhaps wonder how I am able to do this as a profession, they often end their first session by exclaiming that this technique should be part of annual pelvic care because they feel the tremendous positive change in their bodies. Like most bodyworkers, my comfort arises from the professional skill with which I have learned to read and work with body patterns. In approaching the pelvic bowl, rather than focusing on the vagina, I am paying attention to the deeper patterns that run through the whole pelvic bowl: the position of and tension on the ovaries and uterus, the engagement of the pelvic muscles, the tension in myofascial layers (connective tissue that surrounds, supports, and integrates muscles in the body), and the energy patterns that arise during the session.

As a bodyworker, I have learned to see the body holistically. I assess the intricate physical and energetic patterns that travel through the body rather than noticing the body parts themselves. Because women come to my practice by word of mouth, they have faith in this process but still must navigate cultural and even personal hesitation to experience vaginal massage, which is a simplified term for the technique of myofascial release that I am using. As soon as we begin the bodywork process, my clients begin to expand their notion of their bodies. Their hesitation turns to enthusiasm for knowing this part of themselves in a whole new, more holistic and integrated way. To me, this place in the body—where we all begin life—deserves both better care and a true sense of awe for the potential that lies within. My own life has been infinitely enriched by my time spent learning from the pelvic bowl.

Actively engaging or squeezing the muscles around the vagina, which form the pelvic floor, is the first step in assessing pelvic muscular health. This is known as a Kegel exercise: tightening the whole pelvic floor so that these vaginal muscles come together and lift. When one finger is inserted into the vagina, a Kegel feels like a squeeze. As a woman repeats this exercise, I check (touching internally in a circle) each aspect of her pelvic floor for muscle engagement. I divide this circle into four quadrants to assess the top, bottom, right, and left regions of her pelvic floor. Ideally, the muscles are engaging in each quadrant of her pelvic bowl, but typically only part of the pelvic floor is activated. Muscle fibers holding tension and pain (and diminished energy) will have much less movement, or squeezing action, during a Kegel.

Kegels are often prescribed to increase pelvic strength, but I find that they are not beneficial unless a woman's pelvic muscles are already completely engaging, with active movement in each quadrant. Kegels do not change pelvic patterns; they only strengthen the muscles that are free to engage. Most women do not truly have weak pelvic muscles, but rather muscles that are not able to fully engage because of core tension, past traumas, and other pelvic imbalances. The greatest change in a woman's pelvic muscle patterns comes through hands-on vaginal massage, which releases core tension, brings healing, and restores balance so that the root muscles can actively engage. Once pelvic muscles are actively engaging, exercise that strengthens the core further revitalizes the pelvic muscles and Kegels can be a part of a core strengthening program.

Sonya was surprised to learn that even though she had not birthed a baby, her pelvic muscles might be less engaged. I explained that every woman has a range of pelvic motion. As a result of postural patterns, emotional stress, energy blocks, trauma, injuries, or other pelvic events, the pelvic muscles often become imbalanced, meaning one area of muscles tends to do more work than the others. One region or quadrant of the pelvic floor compensates, and the muscles lose their dynamic balance. Over time, muscular imbalances affect a woman's pelvic stability and root health.

While tension in the pelvic muscles restricts the blood and energy flow in a woman's core, supple muscles encourage flow, enhancing overall pelvic and vaginal health. The well-being of a woman's pelvic muscles impacts her level of sensation and plays a vital role in sexual pleasure. When she feels radiant from her center, she carries herself with an inner sense of peace that increases her access to joyful energy. A vibrant pelvic bowl makes a vibrant woman, and taking care of the root supports this vitality.

# The Pelvic Bowl: Your Root Place

To begin your pelvic self-care, it is helpful to visualize your pelvic bowl. This allows you to focus your awareness on the region of your pelvic work. While you may want to find some illustrations to enhance your understanding of pelvic anatomy, in this book I encourage women to sense and feel their bodies, rather than to simply think about them. I have found that the most powerful energetic connections arise from visualizing intuitively and that, by visualizing or sensing, women are more likely to comprehend the full nature of their bodies.

When you begin the process of visualizing, your pelvis may feel like uncharted territory. Simply imagine yourself exploring a unique and largely undiscovered part of your female body that belongs to you alone.

## Visualize the Anatomy of the Pelvic Bowl

The pelvic bowl is your root place in the female body. Bring your attention here when you want to know more about your creative potential or feel the grounding energy of your core.

### Exercise: Visualizing the Anatomy of the Pelvic Bowl

1. First locate the landmarks of your pelvis on your body. Place your hands on the upper boundary of your pelvic bowl, the pelvic crest, sometimes referred to incorrectly as your hips. Move your hands toward the front of your bowl to find your

pubic bone (the bony region in front of your urethra or bladder opening), where the two halves of your pelvis meet. Ponder this connection place. Now move back over the tops of your pelvic bowl and feel how the bones dip down in back. Here the pelvic bones connect with the sacrum, a beautiful triangle-shaped bone that is about the size of your hand and whose tip ends at the coccyx (the tailbone between your buttocks). Place one of your palms over the sacrum and feel the vibrant energy here (there are many nerve endings and blood vessels that weave through the sacrum and nourish the pelvic bowl). These landmarks define the shape of your pelvic bowl. Think about the inner curve of your pelvis and how it forms a protective bowl around your creative center.

2. Close your eyes and imagine your pelvic bowl. Sense the spaciousness within your bowl and notice your inner awareness of this space. You may feel a boundary marked by the bones of your pelvis, but the energy of the bowl is broader than this boundary. Trace the bony boundaries of your pelvis again and sense both the physical and energetic shape of your pelvic bowl.

3. Bring awareness to the deep center of your pelvic bowl, to your uterus. Notice this creative well in your core, a denser energy in the center. What is your connection to this profoundly feminine place and your own internal creative flow? Sense, on either side of your uterus, the radiance of your ovaries (as light or warmth), shining on each side of your bowl. Have you ever noticed this source of inner fire, your own creative sparks?

4. Focus on the base of the pelvis, the pelvic ring. The central structure here, located just below your uterus, is your vagina—

a passageway. The lovemaking that you take into yourself, the blood of your fertility cycle, and any babies you birth vaginally pass through this gateway. Even with cesarean births, energy still releases from the vagina too and can be consciously accessed by breathing and visualizing the birth energy moving through your root. How does your inner vision imagine your vagina? What are you presently releasing or bringing in for your creative core?

5. Picture the base and front of your bowl. On either side of your vaginal opening lie the lips, or labia. Toward the front of your body, as a palpable place of pleasure, is your clitoris. Between your clitoris and vaginal opening is your urethra, and just above the urethra is your bladder. What do you notice in the front of your bowl?

6. Picture the back of your bowl. Toward the back of your root, below your vaginal opening, lies your rectal opening. Between these two openings is your perineum, a dynamic place where many muscle fibers come together. Touching this area provides an immediate sense of grounding, as a place of connection to the earth's energy, and it is involved in the profound expansion that occurs with childbirth. This is also the area that often sustains tears during childbirth, and any scars will benefit from perineal and vaginal massage. Is this dynamic point holding tension or grounding your root?

7. Locate your pubic bone and your coccyx again to mark the front and back of your pelvic ring. Envision a group of muscles covering this entire ring at the base of the pelvis. These vibrant muscles are your pelvic floor, and they provide support to your female organs, maintain your core balance and stability, and play a key role in your sexual

pleasure. Your urethral, vaginal, and rectal openings all pass through your pelvic floor. Make a connection with this base of your pelvis.

8. Find the top of your pubic bone in the front of your pelvis again. Imagine a place just behind it that can be felt through your vagina. This is the famed G-spot, a physical and energy center that can be touched to enhance the sensations of lovemaking. What do you notice when you focus your attention here?

9. Close your visualization and reflect on your observations. Give thanks for this, your precious pelvic bowl.

**Honor the Pelvic Bowl**
What did you notice when visualizing your pelvic bowl? Did you gain an appreciation for the root of your body? Were there any painful feelings regarding your female body or feminine self? Both joyful and challenging pelvic associations have value in restoring root vitality, and each new awareness for your pelvic space increases your connection with this part of your body. Each sense of wounding or pain offers guidance for your healing.

Your pelvis is a powerful base of support; honoring this space will increase its capacity to support you physically, emotionally, and spiritually. The following exercise may assist you to further explore your relationship with your pelvic bowl.

### Exercise: Honoring Your Pelvic Bowl

1. Reflection: Bring awareness to your pelvic bowl and ponder your relationship to your feminine core. Notice how it feels to spend time in your creative center. Acknowledge places in need of healing or celebration.

2. Ritual: Take a piece of paper and spend five minutes writing about your pain or any desires for healing in your pelvic bowl or your relationship to the feminine. On the other side of this paper, write for five minutes about your joy as a woman and your desires for celebration. When you finish, place the paper on your altar or plant it in a garden to honor your pelvic bowl. Each pelvic wound that you begin to heal for yourself and each pelvic appreciation that you find allow you to more joyously embody your feminine form.

## Pelvic Care as Prevention

After receiving a pelvic session, Sonya wanted to know (as so many of my clients do) why more women and healthcare practitioners have not heard of pelvic care. Part of the reason is that the Western medical paradigm rarely emphasizes preventative healthcare. As with many other body systems, pelvic care is typically offered only once a woman has developed significant physical symptoms, like urine leakage or a sensation of heaviness (known as a prolapse) as the uterus moves toward the vaginal opening. Though pelvic care should be part of a woman's healthcare routine, the pelvis is rarely treated preventively, though when it is, imbalances resolve with significantly less effort and time. However, because the standard pelvic care model is symptom-based rather than preventive, many women are unaware of their pelvic imbalances because, initially, they may not show outward symptoms.

Another reason is simply a lack of knowledge regarding pelvic care. Women often suffer silently, without awareness of the available treatments. Others voice their bodily concerns to general healthcare practitioners or family members and are told that their symptoms are a normal result of aging or birthing a child. If women do find their way to a specialist, such as a urologist, most are offered surgery as the main treatment option. Uterine problems are often treated with hysterectomies.

Pelvic symptoms such as pain, urine leakage, or bowel dysfunction can also be embarrassing or feel so shameful that a woman is hesitant to talk about them. She may never learn that she is living with something curable. Women must be persistent in seeking help, because Kegel exercises are often the only tool given in response to pelvic problems. Many healthcare practitioners lack understanding about the need for hands-on and integrative pelvic care to restore core balance. They do not realize that such techniques can change pelvic patterns, and that without them, the body will simply continue its compensation strategies.

A more subtle, but pervasive, reason that pelvic care is unknown is the lack of regard for the female body. The shame associated with the female body may make a woman unconsciously avoid her root, keeping her unaware of the imbalances there. Likewise, most women have pelvic symptoms and imbalances that have been there for so long, they have become accustomed to living with less energy flow in the pelvic bowl. Dampened sensation and energy blocks in the root feel normal. Frequently, after a pelvic care session, my clients are surprised and delighted by the dynamic feeling in their pelvic bowls. Although radiant warmth in the pelvis is a woman's true normal, most have never even experienced their root vitality.

## Make a Pelvic Map

After evaluating the strength of a woman's pelvic muscles, I make a pelvic map by recording, on paper, all her internal points of pelvic tension or pain. Most women have tender areas, or trigger points, in their pelvic muscles even when sexual intercourse is not painful. These are a sign of muscle dysfunction, occurring because a muscle is over- or underused as a result of pelvic imbalances.

Mapping pelvic muscle trigger points aids my understanding of a woman's pelvic pattern and directs the treatment process. With my clients, a pelvic map gives me the information necessary to correct pelvic muscle imbalances with focused vaginal massage. This involves applying pressure and using massage techniques on each tender area. I also guide a woman's awareness to these areas, teaching her to use visualization and breathing exercises to rebalance pelvic muscles by restoring the energy flow. Learning to make a pelvic map is helpful for a woman to understand the tension patterns in her root. In my women's health practice, I teach my clients to locate their own pelvic tension points by using the following exercise.

A pelvic map is made by beginning, internally, at the top of your vagina and touching your internal pelvic region in a clockwise direction, recording any areas of pain or tension, making a complete circle around the pelvic rim. This is a map of the tension, trigger points, and areas of altered sensation in your pelvic muscles. You may find many areas of tenderness or just a few. Initially, locating trigger points will increase your awareness of holding patterns in these root muscles. Working with your points of tension, you can change these patterns to increase the suppleness and health of your root. As you map your pelvic tension points and learn to recognize the internal sensations of this tension, you may also discover how root patterns alert you to the external stresses impacting your feminine core.

### Exercise: Making a Pelvic Map

Read through the exercise first to familiarize yourself with the steps involved. Then find a comfortable and private space to make a pelvic map. You will need a piece of paper and pen and a supported position that allows you access to your vagina. In doing this exercise, you may discover areas of pain or tension as well as a new appreciation of your internal space. You may even be surprised by what you notice—without any particular agenda, simply exploring your body with a curious and open awareness. Do not be concerned if you are unsure about what you are feeling. Over time, when you have become more familiar with your internal landscape, it may be easier to note changes. Also remember that lack of an aware connection with your pelvic bowl makes it difficult for some women to feel much at first and that connection and your feeling can improve with practice.

1. Draw a palm-sized circle on your paper to represent the circular, muscular pelvic floor.

2. Draw an X inside the circle to divide it into four quadrants for mapping—upper (anterior) near your urethral opening, lower (posterior) near your rectal opening, and right and left quadrants.

3. Insert the index finger of one hand into your vagina about one inch, and begin to touch your pelvic muscles near your urethral opening, or the top of your pelvic space. Use gentle touch in this region because just above your urethral opening is your urethra, or tube connecting to the bladder, and it is easily irritated.

4. Begin to feel for areas of tension or pain in your pelvic muscles; these are just like the painful knots found in tight neck or shoulder muscles. Move from the top of your pelvic floor in a clockwise direction. With your other hand, map your findings onto the piece of paper. A small x notes an area of tension, and a big X notes an area of pain. Rate any painful points on a scale of 1 to 10, with 10 as the worst pain. Use an O to indicate areas of decreased sensation.

5. Continue mapping until you have covered the entire circle of your pelvic musculature, touching your internal pelvic muscles point by point by moving around your vagina.

## What to Do with Your Pelvic Map

The pelvic map illustrates the tension patterns in your pelvic bowl, which come from the way that you inhabit your body. First notice the patterns you see. Do you hold tension in a particular quadrant of your pelvic floor? Do you have areas of pain more superficially or deeper in your pelvic muscles? Are there any places of numbness or altered sensation? Compare areas with more tension or pain to those areas with less; how do these regions differ?

When you make a map of your pelvic muscles, you will learn where you tend to carry muscle tension. Though initially marking these points on paper will give you a visual picture of your tension points, it is not necessary to repeat this exercise unless you prefer a visual map. With practice, you can make a mental map of these points just by checking internally once or twice a week. You may find areas that are repeatedly tense, holding chronic tension, while other areas of tension will come and go depending on your overall stress level (just as with tension patterns in the rest of your body).

Tension is the body's means of coping with emotional and physical stress. The tension in your pelvic bowl reveals the stress that is held in your root, but muscles that hold more pain and tension have less elasticity and decreased resilience. These muscles are also less able to engage, weakening your core support. However, working with these points through direct massage, increased awareness, and energy exercises in this book will reengage your pelvic muscles and change these core patterns.

If you have been living with symptoms of pelvic imbalance such as pain, muscle weakness, difficulty doing a Kegel, changes from birthing a baby, or a sense of disconnect from your root, you may also begin to restore function and core balance by working with your pelvic tension points. Releasing chronic muscle tension, reducing your overall stress, and teaching the body how to clear tension even in the presence of stress will significantly enhance the long-term health of your pelvic muscles and organs. Learning to clear the tension in your root allows you to change the structure and holding patterns of your pelvic bowl so they better support your creative center. Seek the assistance of a pelvic care practitioner as needed, but also learn the territory of your own root.

By working with your root tension points on a regular basis, you may also identify sources of chronic root stress such as restrictions in your creative expression or other blocks to your energy flow. These chronic points of tension can be resolved directly through vaginal massage, and also by changing the external situations that repeatedly put stress on your core. Taking care of your root after a stressful event will greatly assist your return to a sense of well-being. The following story illustrates how to use a pelvic map in this manner.

### Women's Stories: The Pelvic Floor as Personal Gauge

Laura came for pelvic work to address a chronic pattern of hemorrhoids, a common pelvic floor discomfort that often goes untreated due to lack of awareness about pelvic care. Laura's pelvic map revealed multiple areas of tension and tenderness in the posterior region of her pelvic floor muscles, near her tailbone and rectum. Tension in this area of the pelvic floor often results in physical problems such as hemorrhoids, constipation, and tailbone or coccyx pain. Posterior pelvic dysfunction may require rectal massage (another way to alleviate root tension) as well as vaginal massage to restore pelvic balance. Laura also had an area of numbness in her left pelvic floor region.

With pelvic massage to alleviate muscle tension and focused breathing exercises to restore energy flow, I helped Laura reduce the tension and pain in her posterior pelvic floor and increase the sensation in her left pelvic musculature. Laura learned how to make a pelvic map and practice vaginal self-massage, ending the first session with a balanced and relaxed pelvic space.

Over the next several weeks, Laura monitored and mapped her pelvic muscles' response to various experiences. The most frequent correlation she discovered was that any type of conflict caused increased pelvic pain and tension; the more upsetting the conflict, the higher the level of irritation in her pelvic muscles—both in the number of tender areas and in the intensity of the pain. An argument with her partner and a subsequent disagreement with her boss produced similar pelvic maps and a recurrence of hemorrhoids. Laura's body's response revealed that she was more upset than she had realized.

When I confirmed that unresolved conflicts create body tension, Laura shared an experience of her own pelvic selfcare. While working on her body, she was thinking about her desire to start her own business and felt her pelvic muscles relax. Laura knew that she looked to both her partner and her boss for support, but they never seemed to validate her needs. In her body's response, Laura found that she desired new modes of support for herself.

Posterior pelvic tension often indicates that a woman's needs for support are not being met in the way that her spirit longs for. Sometimes the support needed is emotional, other times physical. She may need a new form of partnership, more self-care, a particular creative outlet, or a transition in some aspect of her life. As each woman begins to examine and create the support she seeks, she will find a greater sense of ease and balance in her posterior pelvic floor.

Several months later, Laura told me that she had launched her own business. Because of her new business responsibilities and the external stress involved with them, she guessed that her pelvis would hold more tension, but her pelvic map was actually healthier, with almost no tension in the pelvic muscles and very few painful areas. She also noticed more sensation when touching her left vaginal muscles.

Laura explained that she had always wanted to work for herself. In retrospect, she realized that working for someone else had created substantial stress that she held internally, which was clear in her pelvic map. Once she decided to live more freely, her body seemed to let go of this tension. She stopped looking for validation from a boss or her partner, both external sources, and discovered that providing for herself gave her the type of support she was seeking. Laura would never have predicted that starting her own business might create a relaxed pelvic space, but her pelvic map provided a direct gauge of her experience.

As she created the support she desired, Laura also found more freedom in her body and life. Mapping her pelvic floor provided a clear picture of how this change in personal choices reduced the core stress and enhanced the vitality of her pelvic space.

## Numbness: Recover Your Hope

When exploring the root of the female body, some women encounter regions of dampened sensation or disconnection. Numbness can be a decrease in actual physical sensation or an emotional numbness that causes a woman to lose her focus when she brings her awareness to a particular region of her pelvic bowl. A sensation of numbness typically indicates a pelvic separation or disassociation resulting from physical or emotional trauma. Even a hard fall to the tailbone can disrupt the alignment of the pelvic bowl and set up patterns of pelvic disassociation.

Pelvic disassociations are part of the body's defense mechanism. They serve as a protective response to an overwhelming experience. Still, once a traumatic event is over, these places of separation limit a woman's access to her feminine wisdom and maintain imbalances in the pelvis. When a woman encounters an area of numbness in her pelvic bowl, it signals an opportunity to restore her pelvic presence and heal any separation between her female body and feminine spirit.

Rediscovering these areas of numbness or disassociation may initially involve listening for past experiences of pain. As you begin, proceed at your own pace and gather your resources. Do your pelvic work and access your feelings slowly; then let yourself process and integrate each new sensation or awareness. The female body is your feminine ground. Wherever your numbness is, whether in emotional expression, pelvic sensation, or the energy of your womb space, the healing potential is there as well. Look for regions of lost ground, actions you turn away from unconsciously—taking up your rightful space, protecting or caring for yourself, cultivating your creativity, or expressing your sensuality—and restore your presence in each place. Reflections for areas of numbness include:

Where in your body do you have difficulty finding your
awareness?
What support do you need to re-access your ability to feel?
Where in your life do you notice places of numbness or
shutdown?
How can you recover your hope and presence in these regions?

## Restore Your Pelvic Presence

Your pelvic presence is an energetic quality—it indicates the level of connection you have with your root. A strong pelvic presence allows you to clear energetic debris and identify energetic imbalances. A solid presence actively engages the root of your body and conveys an intention to hold your feminine ground.

To increase your pelvic presence, bring your attention to your core on a regular basis. Notice the quality of energy or sensations that you find. The quality of energy in your root will impact the energy that you draw into your life. Taking a moment each day to clarify your pelvic energy restores your active presence in this vital place and heals previous disruptions.

### Exercise: Clarifying the Energy of Your Bowl

1. Assess your pelvic energy by focusing on the sensations of your root. If you feel at ease or peaceful in your center, the energy is clear. If you feel agitated, negative, tense, or have difficulty keeping your focus, it is time to clarify the energy.

2. Walk the edges of your bowl with your inner awareness, starting in front and moving to the right. Traveling along the full perimeter, imagine lightly sweeping and touching each place. Visualize an element (like air, water, or fire) cleansing your bowl, balancing the energy, and assisting the movement of stagnant energy down through your root and into the earth.

3. Pay particular attention to any areas of your bowl that you might tend to avoid and work in those areas with focused intent. Your bowl is not dirty, but simply in need of attention. Clarify your bowl with love and respect, using gentle and thoughtful movements.

4. When you are finished, bless your pelvic bowl by calling in the radiant energy of the universe. Imagine the golden warmth of sunlight touching and filling your center.

### Women's Stories: Reclaiming Her Pelvic Space

Camilla was interested in pelvic work for connecting with her vagina and pelvis, but she had difficulty feeling or tightening her pelvic muscles. She said that her pelvis did not even feel like a part of her body.

Camilla had been sexually abused as a child, and as a result her vagina and pelvis did not feel safe to her. As an adult, she had worked through many of the emotional aspects of this trauma, and now she wanted to reconnect more intentionally with this part of her body.

Initially, maintaining her focus in the pelvic space felt overwhelming as she encountered the parts of her muscles that were still associated with past abuse. I encouraged her to feel the sensations of her muscles reawakening and to direct her breath to each region she noticed, to assist her body's ability to integrate new sensory information. Between our sessions, she worked with a counselor and actively nurtured herself to process the emotions arising with pelvic contact. With a combination of physical and emotional tools, she found the right pace to proceed with working on her body.

Camilla realized that she had never become aware of her vagina on her own terms before someone else seemed to claim it. She had formed her feminine identity without a sense of ownership regarding her female body, so in first bringing attention to her pelvic space, she initially found almost no sensation or body awareness in this region.

She recognized that her pelvic numbness helped her avoid the pain that was held there. But she knew she was missing her joy as well. To reconnect with her body, Camilla had to travel through layers of feelings: fear, rage, sadness, and grief. With each step, she reclaimed more sensation and awareness of her own energy in her vagina and pelvic bowl. She eventually took back this precious part of herself.

## The Rewards of Pelvic Care

After a few sessions of pelvic rebalancing, I teach my clients to do pelvic self-care. Every woman can learn how to actively engage her pelvic muscles, change pelvic tension patterns, and identify sources of tension in her life that create imbalances in her core. By discovering how to care for the female body, a woman establishes a new relationship with her feminine self.

As the root place of the female body, the pelvic bowl contains the richness of each woman's experiences. When you look into your own pelvic patterns and bring awareness to your root, expect no less than to encounter your feminine self in the truth of her wounds and beauty, especially as you learn one of the essential tools for pelvic self-care: the practice of vaginal massage.

## Vaginal Massage: The Way to a Vibrant Root

A nonsexual internal massage that soothes and invigorates a woman's core muscles, vaginal massage is a vital tool for women's health physical therapists in alleviating pelvic symptoms, and it is an essential part of restoring physical and energetic balance to the pelvic bowl. By applying general massage techniques to the internal vagina, this kind of massage reaches the core pelvic muscles commonly holding pelvic tension. Vaginal massage is more nourishing than sexual because it works on the deep internal muscles of the pelvic bowl, rather than on the sensory-rich skin or clitoris.

I teach vaginal self-massage to women to offer them a new way to take care of themselves. Most women have only associated the root of their body with sex, or possibly childbirth, and some have never even touched their own vagina or internal pelvic space. Ideally all women should know both how to pleasure themselves sexually and also how to nourish the root with vaginal massage. The root of the female body is a precious place; self-care is meant to be joyful and honoring. If a woman finds that she is hesitant to do vaginal massage or otherwise apply pelvic self-care, working through this resistance is part of her healing process.

## Addressing Pelvic Tension

Pelvic muscles play a key role in a woman's overall structural support system, sense of relaxation, and ability to experience sexual pleasure. All these functions are inhibited by pelvic tension, which can be released with vaginal massage.

Though pelvic tension interferes with a woman's ability to use her pelvic floor muscles in daily activities, the body compensates to the best of its abilities, attempting to provide core support even with limited function. The body copes with a pelvic imbalance until something (injury, pelvic trauma, childbirth, stress, or the hormonal changes of menopause) prevents the pelvic muscles from continuing to compensate. Then a woman may begin to experience the more severe pelvic symptoms (like pain, organ prolapse, or urine leakage) that result from these long-term pelvic imbalances.

Vaginal massage addresses pelvic imbalances before symptoms arise and should be a part of every woman's self-care. After a session of vaginal massage, women tell me that they have a completely new awareness of their pelvic bowl and vagina. With vaginal massage softening their core, women say they have never felt so deeply relaxed or centered.

## How to Do Vaginal Self-Massage

Use a pelvic map, or your own internal sensation, to direct your massage to the areas of pain and tension in your pelvic muscles. The objective of vaginal massage is to increase your connection and awareness for this part of your body. The places in our bodies where we have better awareness often correlate to increased blood and energy flow, ultimately enhancing cellular health. Rather than trying to do something specific with your massage, instead work to increase your respectful connection to your pelvic muscles. Just the act of touch alone will enhance your body awareness.

The following exercise describes the process of vaginal self-massage for a woman taking care of herself (it is not meant as a description for practitioners). Caution: Vaginal self-massage should not be attempted while pregnant or until at least eight weeks postpartum.

### Exercise: Vaginal Self-Massage

Find a comfortable and private place and a position that allows you to easily access your vagina.

1. Lie on your side with your legs apart and slightly bent. Insert your index finger or thumb into your vagina and touch your pelvic muscles by moving your finger over to the sides of your vaginal opening. Use gentle pressure and pay attention to the response of your body. You can touch areas simply to focus awareness or you can smooth the muscle fibers in a basic massage stroke. Do not massage the area over your urethra (at the front of your pelvic bowl) or your rectum (at the bottom of your pelvic bowl); these areas are very sensitive and require light touch.

2. The first few times, just become familiar with the sensations of your internal pelvis. Try to touch and notice, rather than attempt to change, the areas of tension in your pelvic bowl. Use light strokes (as if smoothing or sculpting the muscles), moving your finger from the front of your internal pelvis to the back on each side, or deep pressure on specific trigger points, whatever your body enjoys. Listen to your body. When you feel ready, slow your breathing and soften each area of tension by increasing your connection to this area while you massage. You do not need to release all the tension; releasing even a fraction will begin changing your core patterns of pelvic muscular imbalance.

3. Make either circular movements or hold steady pressure on any areas of pain or tension. Follow along the internal rim of your pelvic bowl (by feeling for the hardness of your pelvis) and massage this region just inside your vaginal opening. You may work on the tender areas that you found in your pelvic map or others that you encounter while exploring.

4. Move deeper inside your vagina and to either side toward your internal hip joints (an area that commonly holds pelvic tension).

5. Finish your massage and give thanks for the root of your female body.

**Frequently Asked Questions About Vaginal Self-Massage**

The best way to do vaginal self-massage is to listen to your own body and to do what feels right. However, as you develop your technique, answers to these common questions may assist you:

**What am I trying to do?** Rather than achieving a particular outcome, you are establishing a loving relationship with your body. You are becoming familiar with your own internal pelvic bowl and learning how to read and communicate with your core. With hands-on massage, you are soothing your body. Bodies respond to touch, and respectful and loving touch can change and enrich your root patterns. By working with your root, you will support your body in realigning with core balance as its norm.

**What are the benefits of vaginal massage?** Vaginal massage increases your sense of peace and deep relaxation because it reduces tension and increases cellular flow in a central region of your body. It improves your overall pelvic muscular health, strength, and vitality, enabling these muscles to enhance their function as your core structural support. By encouraging the physical well-being of your pelvis, you become more energetically present in your pelvic bowl and able to access the energy resources it contains. You may also notice increased sensation and muscular tone in your vagina, as well as enhanced sexual arousal and enjoyment.

**How often and for how long should I do vaginal massage?** If you are healing from pelvic pain or a particular pelvic event (childbirth, miscarriage, medical procedure, or period of increased stress) or just reestablishing a connection to your root, two to three sessions a week may be necessary. Self-care sessions may range from five minutes to a half hour, based on your available time and pelvic needs. The support you give your root will increase your ability to receive energy and restore balance in the midst of challenging experiences. Doing vaginal massage on a regular basis will encourage new patterns that bring vitality to your core. As a maintenance program, one to two sessions per month are fine. Take note if you begin feeling edgy, tense, or easily irritated; this is a sign that your pelvic floor is holding too much tension, blocking your energy flow, and in need of a massage. Pelvic symptoms such as heaviness, prolapse, urine leakage, or recurrent pain signal that your pelvic muscles require rebalancing from a pelvic specialist.

**What if I feel awkward?** Keep trying. The root is an essential part of your body, with valuable energy and resources for you as a woman. You deserve to feel at ease with caring for this place. If you can rub the sore spots in your shoulders, you can rub the sore spots in your root. Try to feel and sense, working on the root through your sensations and body awareness rather than thinking about it or questioning what you feel with your mind. Even touching your root with thoughtful regard and directing your breath there will enable your core connection. Learning how to clear tension in your core and connecting more deeply with your root will greatly enhance your creative flow, your sense of joy, your ability to clear blocks and restore core balance, and your awe for what your female body does for you.

**What position should I be in?** Experiment until you find a position that allows you to reach your pelvic muscles and be comfortable enough to relax your body. Positions may include side-lying, propped with pillows, sitting in the bathtub, or even standing in the shower. You may reach down between your legs or lie on your side and reach from behind. Finding an ideal position and refining your massage technique may mean feeling awkward for a while, but just as you take care of other parts of your body, you will be able to take care of your root with practice and patience.

**How far should I put my finger into my vagina?** You may massage very superficially or on the sides of your internal pelvis as far as you can reach; areas of pain and tension may be shallow or deep. You may use your index finger or thumb, whatever works for you. Try to find pelvic tension anywhere in or around your vaginal opening.

**How hard should I press?** Your pressure will change depending on your body's response. Use as much pressure on the muscle as required to release tension. If your pelvic tension begins to increase or you feel your body beginning to guard rather than relax, decrease your pressure or stop the session altogether. Your body may be signaling that it has had enough. Again, use very gentle pressure near the urethra and rectum. Think of your touch as sculpting your pelvic muscles, sometimes light, other times firm, but always moving in smooth lines and working together with your body.

**What if I don't notice any particular pain, weakness, or numbness? Am I doing it wrong?** No, sometimes the root massage is more energetic than physical, and instead of physical changes, you feel energy moving and a state of relaxation like you might experience in a meditation. Images or thoughts may come to mind, you may visualize colors or light, or you may become aware of different sensations in your body. You are expanding your ability to connect with the vibrant and healing energy of your creative center.

**What if I feel a pulsing sensation or heat as I massage?** These are normal signs of muscular and energetic release, indicating an increased blood and energy flow, and decreased tension. This is just what you want to feel as your pelvic vitality returns.

**Is vaginal massage ever sexually arousing?** Vaginal massage is quite different from sexual stimulation and typically feels more like the relaxation experienced with regular body massage. Also, the release experienced by sex and orgasm is more focal and temporary while the release obtained from vaginal massage can be felt throughout the pelvic bowl (even into the belly) and tends to be sustained. (*Note*: Sex also supports pelvic health because it massages the inner pelvis and invigorates a woman's pelvic energy and blood flow, but it does not address or change long-term pelvic patterns of imbalance.) The vagina is most typically associated with sexuality, but it is helpful to recognize the vagina as more than a sexual place. It is the primary entry to the pelvic bowl and a woman's own access to the root of her body. To be able to do vaginal massage, a woman may encounter her associations with sexuality—and if she has negative associations, she might have to change these in order to take care of her root. Releasing muscle tension in the core with vaginal massage often leads to enhanced sensation and greater potential for orgasm during sexual intercourse because of the increased blood and energy flow available in a relaxed pelvic floor.

**I am surprised to find many painful areas in my pelvic muscles; why are they there?** Painful areas, or trigger points, occur in muscles that have chronic tension and are most common in core regions like the jaw, neck, back, hips, and pelvic area. These core regions are particularly sensitive to the chronic tension that arises from emotional or physical stress. When a muscle has chronic tension, it builds up lactic acid and other cellular debris. The tension constricts the vessels, inhibiting the in- and outflow that maintain a healthy muscle. Stress patterns tend to be maintained by imbalances in posture, prolonged sitting, or habits of daily living. Trigger points are always worse when stress increases, but they can be completely resolved by increasing root muscle health with vaginal massage, restoring core balance, and creating a life of balance to diminish overall stress.

**What if a painful spot becomes more painful as I massage?** Applying direct pressure to painful spots (trigger points) in a muscle is a standard massage technique. As you push on this area, the pain will initially increase. But then, as pressure is sustained, the pain will typically dissipate as the muscle softens and releases its tension. This is a useful technique to change patterns of pelvic muscular tension and enhance overall blood and energy flow to the muscle. In applying this technique, pay attention to your general body tension. Pain causes a contraction response in the body. If you can breathe toward the pain and continue to relax your body as you apply direct pressure to a trigger point, then increasing pain prior to a release is fine. If, however, you apply pressure for several minutes with no change in muscle tension, or your general body tension begins to increase, give your pelvic muscles a break.

**Where should I begin if I have several painful spots?** When pelvic muscles have many painful areas, vaginal massage may initially seem overwhelming or even produce a feeling of nausea. This is because these pelvic muscles are in real distress and in need of attention. If this pattern is not addressed, your pelvic health will suffer. Start slowly and use your pelvic care tools. Drink plenty of water and get lots of rest after each session, because your body will flush the built-up toxins. Incorporate more movement into your daily routine; static postures tend to increase pelvic stagnation. Place a warm cloth or hot water bottle on your low belly or perineum if sore. Use a holistic approach to identify and change external patterns contributing to pelvic imbalances; you will feel better.

**Will I be sore afterward?** After doing a vaginal massage and releasing core tension, you may be sore or experience a cramping sensation in your pelvic muscles for a few hours or a day. This can be normal as the tension clears and the body learns how to integrate the new core pattern. Prolonged soreness beyond a day means that too much was done in one session (either too many points or too much time). Soothe sore muscles with a warm bath and in your next vaginal massage session, use a lighter touch or do less overall.

**What if an area of tension does not release?** Sometimes a particular area of tension is not ready to release. If you encounter this, try working on a different region of your pelvis. You might ask your body what it is holding or what it needs to be able to release the tension. Remember that even a small change in your level of pelvic tension will begin to shift your pelvic patterns. In the case of vaginal massage, more is not necessarily better. Doing too much at once may actually set you back by overloading your body's ability to integrate the new muscular pattern you are creating. Continue your massage as long as you obtain muscular release; when your pelvic muscles stop releasing, end the session.

**How do I know if I am making a change?** Several things may indicate a positive change in your pelvic muscles. Look for decreased muscle tension; for example, your finger may be able to press into the muscle more deeply or the muscle will soften. Notice an overall increase in your sense of relaxation; perhaps you are taking deeper breaths or feeling at ease in your body. The painful sensation in a tender place may decrease or resolve completely. Your ability to engage your pelvic muscles may increase in one or more quadrants. Squeeze your vaginal muscles around your finger to discover changes in pelvic muscle movement—the pelvic muscles may engage more smoothly and evenly. Sense the energy flow in your pelvis: it may feel more expansive or vibrant.

**I am pregnant and want to prepare my body for birth. Can I do vaginal massage?** My philosophy while someone is pregnant is to leave the nest alone and not attempt to change core patterns with vaginal massage. Touching yourself (or making love with your partner) with respect and tenderness will increase blood flow and provide nourishment to the pelvic muscles in preparation for birth. I wait to begin vaginal massage until six to eight weeks postpartum, and the pelvic bowl exhibits tremendous healing potential with good support. Women should have no fear about the root in regard to birth, because with hands-on pelvic massage to assist their postpartum healing and pelvic alignment, they will often feel more vibrant than before the birth of their baby.

**I recently gave birth vaginally and my pelvic muscles feel weak and stretched. Will vaginal massage help me?** Yes! Vaginal massage is a tremendous support for your body after childbirth, both to assist its healing and completely restore balance to the muscles of the pelvic bowl. Wait at least eight weeks postpartum, after you have stopped bleeding, to do your own internal massage. Within a day of birthing, you may do gentle pelvic squeezes (about 10 to 15 per day) to remind the muscles how to engage after the profound opening of birth. Likewise, visualize and notice the sensations of your pelvic bowl to deepen your awareness for the energy that accompanies each birth event. The most important tool for restoring your body's resources and protecting pelvic health is to rest—lying down several times a day, lifting nothing heavier than your baby, and giving yourself frequent nourishment.

**I find myself avoiding my pelvic region. Would you recommend vaginal massage?** It is difficult to bring awareness to a part of your body that is associated with grief or any pain, but you will find healing if you are able to do so. For example, when a woman has a miscarriage, she may have difficulty reconnecting to the part of her body associated with loss. Miscarriage is a birth event (but not always recognized as such)—and just as with birth, the body needs to rest and recover. Vaginal massage supports this process and also assists a woman in reconnecting with her root to receive the energy and blessings of each birth event. Likewise, any time a woman associates the pelvic bowl with shame, whether because of sexual abuse or other past traumas, a woman may avoid her root. But her greatest healing arises from reclaiming this place for herself. Gathering the necessary providers to help her begin a process of reconnection—and adding vaginal massage or other means of self-care—is all part of this healing journey.

**I had a cesarean birth but still feel different in my pelvic area. Should I do vaginal massage?** Even with a cesarean birth, the pelvic muscles, vagina, and fascia (a layer of tissue that covers the muscles and organs) can become stretched either from the pregnancy or the force required to lift a baby from the uterus. The stretch alters the position of the uterus in the pelvic bowl and decreases the ability of pelvic muscles to engage. Vaginal massage restores balance in the core by assisting these muscles in reengaging and by supporting the uterus in returning to its proper position. If the birth event felt traumatic in any way, vaginal massage also helps you to reconnect with your root and heal on a deeper level.

**I have a scar in my perineum from tearing (and receiving stitches) with childbirth. The scar still feels tight and painful six months later. Will vaginal massage change this?** Any scar in the body can become more flexible and less painful with massage, including a cesarean scar. In this case, it helps to do vaginal massage to alleviate tension in the pelvic muscles, which may be adding to the tension in the scar or inhibiting blood flow. Then also massage the perineum and scar directly with castor oil or vitamin E. No matter how long you have had a scar, massage will increase its suppleness (also increasing blood and energy flow). Your root will feel so much better.

**Is there a specific technique for addressing hemorrhoids?** Hemorrhoids are typically an indication of lower (posterior) quadrant pelvic tension or result from the stretching that accompanies childbirth. Massage the posterior quadrant of your pelvic muscles vaginally, just to the left and right of your rectum. Also, many pelvic providers supplement the treatment process with rectal massage by applying direct pressure to painful areas at the rectal opening and about a quarter inch inside the rectum. These points may be quite sensitive, but sustained pressure applied to them will often bring significant release to the pelvic muscles and resolve the hemorrhoids. The other reason that hemorrhoids appear, besides posterior quadrant tension, is that the posterior quadrant is actually working too hard because of an imbalance elsewhere in the pelvic muscles. Therefore, generalized vaginal massage may also bring relief from hemorrhoids.

**I do my vaginal massage, but my pelvic tension keeps returning. What should I do?** Vaginal massage changes root tension patterns over time, and these tension patterns are found in layers. You may be discovering deeper layers of tension that have been there for many years. Keep doing your massage on a regular basis, and each layer of tension will dissolve. You will notice your progress because you are able to tolerate a deeper or longer massage, and your tension (or painful areas) will dissolve more quickly in response to your touch. With repetition, your pelvic muscles will soften even in response to your breath (focused breathing restores energy flow) because they have established the pathway to a more relaxed and supple root. Look for and change external sources of stress that may be contributing to root tension and also address emotional energies that convey unmet needs.

**When should I seek professional assistance?** If you discover pelvic muscle imbalances that persist during self-care sessions, additional help is needed. You may also want to seek outside guidance simply to learn from a professional and refine your pelvic techniques. Enlist the support of a women's health physical therapist or pelvic care specialist whenever you experience pelvic symptoms such as urine leakage, pelvic pain, prolapse, or a feeling of pelvic heaviness. Additionally, it is beneficial to seek professional care to address pelvic trauma related to difficult childbirth, miscarriage, a fall impacting your tailbone, abuse, surgery, or another major pelvic experience. After birthing a child, you may feel intimidated by the changes in your body. Likewise, the grief held in your root after a miscarriage, birth loss, or other pelvic trauma may be overwhelming. Working on your own body will still make you feel better; touch in the root is grounding and assists your body's capacity to move energy. Receiving pelvic care from a practitioner simply provides another source of external support.

## Women's Stories: Addressing Pelvic Imbalances Preventatively

Erin came for pelvic work after a friend told her about my practice of pelvic care. She and her partner wanted to have a child, and she thought that her body would benefit from pelvic work before getting pregnant. She had never experienced any pelvic problems and did not expect that I would find much to work on. Still, she thought that receiving pelvic care would be valuable.

Erin's pelvic map surprised her. It showed decreased strength in all her pelvic quadrants as well as multiple areas of tension and pain. She did not have painful sex and would not have guessed that there were so many painful places in her vaginal muscles, so she asked me what might have caused this.

I explained that Erin's pelvic map, with its multiple trigger points, was fairly typical with prolonged pelvic imbalances. As the result of long-term habits, previous traumas, or everyday stresses, the pelvic muscles begin to function in an imbalanced way. Only some of the muscle fibers remain active; the others hold tension or have difficulty engaging. Over time, the active fibers become strong but overutilized, while the inactive fibers become weak and inaccessible. Tender places in the muscle and chronic patterns of tension are signs of these muscular imbalances.

Erin was fortunate to be addressing her pelvic muscular imbalances prior to pregnancy and childbirth. The earlier a woman resolves her pelvic imbalances, the more easily they are changed. True, I have seen changes in the muscular patterns of women in their seventies and eighties who have birthed eight to ten children, so it is never too late. Still, I want women to have the knowledge and access to pelvic care as early and as often as possible.

After a session of vaginal massage, Erin was able to actively tighten her pelvic muscles with a much stronger squeeze, and she was excited to feel her vaginal muscles respond when she tightened them. She demonstrated an increased vaginal response after the massage, because a relaxed muscle is able to engage, or squeeze and release, across a greater range than a tense muscle.

Carrying tension in your pelvic muscles is like trying to pick up an item when your arms are already full: you simply have no room for anything else. If you set something down, however, you have additional capacity. Likewise, if your pelvic muscles are tense, you cannot actively tighten them because they are already being used. But if you decrease the pain and tension in your pelvic muscles with vaginal massage, they will be more available to respond when you need them.

## Engage Your Core Vitality

Engaging core vitality means accessing the full range of your pelvic muscles. These muscles can be tightened to create a coming-together sensation (squeeze) or fully released to make an opening sensation. Think of a flower to visualize the movements of the pelvic muscles surrounding the vagina: completely closed to symbolize a tightening and fully open to symbolize a release. When you visualize the beauty and range of movement in a flower that opens and closes its petals, you will appreciate the potential in the muscles of the vagina.

Typically women are taught only one aspect of this range: the Kegel exercise, which actively tightens the vaginal muscles. This is the same vaginal squeezing action that a woman with well-developed pelvic tone may use with her partner during sex. However, while the squeeze tends to be emphasized, both ends of the range—engaging and releasing—serve a vital purpose in a woman's vaginal health.

Full tightening of the vaginal muscles from all four pelvic quadrants creates a dynamic lifting sensation. If you are sitting, tighten your pelvic muscles; you can feel them lift your vagina away from the chair. Frequently, the pelvic muscles engage in an unbalanced manner. With only part of the pelvic muscles engaging, the pelvic squeeze is uncoordinated and rough. If the whole base of the pelvic floor engages evenly, then a pelvic squeeze feels like a smooth and fluid lift. After engaging your muscles, now release them, as if exhaling and letting go of all muscular tension in your core. This full release of the pelvic floor allows the muscles to rest and restore themselves. Restoration of pelvic muscles is essential preparation for more dynamic movement.

Tension in the vaginal muscles is commonly mistaken for tone or strength. A tight pelvic floor may actually be the result of high muscle tension or guarding, a sign of muscular imbalance and dysfunction. Well-toned muscles are able to access their full range from resting to dynamically engaging. Tense muscles, on the other hand, hold continuously and have little or no movement when a woman tries to actively engage them. When she clears her pelvic tension and muscular imbalances preventively, a woman is able to access her full vaginal range on a daily basis and receive this core support.

## Evaluate Your Pelvic Engagement

Think of engaging your pelvic muscles as a graceful and restorative movement to nourish your root rather than as a should-do exercise.

Doing a few thoughtful pelvic muscle squeezes through your full vaginal range brings energy and blood flow to your core. Instead of intensity, look for balance and motion in your vaginal squeeze, with all quadrants engaging across their full range. Rather than simply focusing on strength, the key to a healthy pelvic floor is being able to engage the pelvic muscles in a balanced manner. If you find that your pelvic engagement is unbalanced, do a session of vaginal massage and work with your pelvic patterns to restore your whole root capacity. Evaluate your vaginal movement with the following exercise.

### Exercise: Evaluating Your Pelvic Engagement

Find a comfortable and private place and a standing position that allows you to easily access your vagina.

1. Engage your pelvic muscles. While standing, insert your index finger into your vagina and actively squeeze your pelvic muscles. You should feel a squeeze all the way around your finger from each region of your pelvic muscles. Feel the movement of each quadrant and how, together, they tighten in the shape of a ring. Notice which areas of this pelvic ring are engaging strongly and which areas have little or no movement: A *strong* pelvic region will move toward the center and then lift, producing a squeeze with even pressure all around your finger. An *active* pelvic region will move toward the center but not lift, producing an uneven squeeze but still noticeable movement to your finger. A *weak* pelvic region will have little to no movement. If you are having trouble feeling any muscle movement, try lying down to see if this changes your ability to engage your pelvic muscles. Typically, standing is the most challenging position because your pelvic muscles are lifting against gravity.

2. Release your pelvic muscles. When you release your pelvic muscles, notice if any tension remains. Feel the solid structure of your pelvic bones and rest your pelvic muscles against this support. Allow the center of your female body to rest completely. Muscles are designed to engage and then rest. Exhale and let go of any extra holding in your root muscles or pelvic bowl. From the center of your bowl, let the relaxation spread through your body, like circles of vibrant energy radiating out from the core.

3. Address vaginal movement imbalances. Ideally, all regions of the pelvic muscles will strongly engage and then fully release. Try massaging a less responsive region to see if your pelvic movement pattern changes. Continue your vaginal massage sessions or seek the care of a pelvic provider to further address any imbalances you discover. Give thanks to these vital muscles for supporting your female body.

**Learn Your Pelvic Tension Points**
When you evaluate your vaginal muscles, pay attention to pain or reduced movement in the quadrants of your pelvic floor. These are your regions of pelvic tension, and because they hold tension, these areas are unavailable for dynamic muscle function. Familiarize yourself with these places and direct your vaginal massage there.

In my work with pelvic tension, I have noticed that the patterns often correspond to greater themes in a woman's life. Ultimately, changing chronic tension patterns involves identifying the sources of her pelvic tension. By paying attention to what causes her root tension, a woman can consciously reduce the stress in her life.

Listen to your own body's wisdom and make the changes that are meaningful for you. Making the personal changes that serve your well-being will be most beneficial in reducing tension and supporting the vitality of your root.

## Anterior-Quadrant Pelvic Tension: Where Is Your Fear?

In Oriental medicine, the bladder is associated with the emotion of fear, and with my clients as well, tender points near the urethra often signify issues relating to fear. Although many women hold fear in this region, the reasons are unique to each woman. Reflections about top-quadrant pelvic tension include:

What are you holding in the tension of your anterior pelvis?
What fears do you have regarding your female body or creative vitality?
How would you live if you released these fears?

### Women's Stories: Working with Her Fear

Deborah had a frequent burning sensation in her urethra, but tests for a bladder infection came back negative. (Sometimes tension in the anterior pelvic floor produces a change in urinary sensations, but other problems, like infection, must be ruled out first.)

Deborah had multiple anterior-quadrant points of tension, and as I massaged the tension in these muscles, they became hot to the touch. I asked Deborah if she could feel the heat as the tension released. She felt it, but she also felt intense fear. In sensing her fear, Deborah's breathing became shallow and her pelvic energy froze. I encouraged her to bring awareness back to her pelvic bowl. As she did so, the pelvic energy began to flow again and her breath normalized.

Deborah was unclear about the cause of her fear. I explained that the pelvis often holds tension when we routinely compromise ourselves in some way and that working with the tension can also bring up hidden feelings and teach us how to take better care of ourselves. I described the pelvic map and how she might use it to understand her tension patterns. By observing the changes in her pelvic tension and sensing her core energy, Deborah could learn about the sources of external stress contributing to a particular pelvic pattern.

Deborah returned two weeks later to report her findings. She was involved in a new relationship, but she always had difficulty becoming sexually active with her partners. It had been several years since she had last had sex, and she was both nervous and excited about the potential of exploring her sexuality again.

During her pelvic mapping, she noticed a significant increase in pelvic tension on two occasions: once after she and her partner had sex, and a second time after they shared some of their feelings about their developing relationship. Deborah found that on both occasions, she was afraid that her partner would leave if she expressed any of her own needs. Again, she noticed a tendency for her core energy to freeze in the presence of her fear, but by focusing on her pelvic bowl rather than on her fear, she was able to restore her energy flow. Deborah recognized a similar pattern with previous partners and even friends, and it prevented her from having the intimate connections she craved.

By observing her pelvic response, Deborah became more aware of her internal freezing response and the tendency to ignore her own needs. Because she could only deny these needs for a limited time, she often avoided establishing intimate relationships. With a greater awareness of her pelvic bowl, though, she began to use the tension in her body and the sense of holding her energy in as a signal that she needed to acknowledge and even give voice to these needs. In this way, she stopped her pattern of self-denial and resolved the chronic tension in her root. Deborah found that her pelvic muscles still sometimes tightened when she felt vulnerable. But instead of tightening her muscles or freezing in fear, she brought awareness and breath to her center and paid attention to her own needs until she felt her body relax.

Fear can be protective, but living in fear limits your creative energy flow and ability to live fully. Acknowledge your fears and work with them directly to release the tension in your anterior pelvic bowl and embody your true potential.

## Left-Quadrant Pelvic Tension: What Are You Receiving?

Tension in the left quadrant of the pelvic muscles often relates to a woman's receiving something into her body or life that creates conflict within her feminine self. The left quadrant has tension patterns similar to those that arise with energetic imbalances in the left ovary because the left side is typically the more feminine or receptive region of the body (more information about the feminine versus masculine aspects of the body is in chapter 4). Reflections regarding left-quadrant pelvic tension include:

What are you holding in the tension of the left side of your pelvis?

What are you receiving that you would rather not?

What would your life look like if you honored your own wishes?

### Women's Stories: Learning to Honor Herself

Maria sought pelvic care to strengthen her pelvic muscles. She was unable to sustain some of her core yoga exercises and noticed a feeling of air passing (like vaginal gas) through her muscles (a sign of pelvic imbalance) and a general disconnect to her pelvic space while attempting them. Her pelvic map revealed multiple areas of tension and tenderness in the left pelvic quadrant. Maria's pelvic tension was minimally responsive to vaginal massage, indicating a strong external component maintaining this pelvic pattern.

I told Maria that her body did not seem ready to release this particular pelvic tension, and then I taught her the self-release and pelvic mapping techniques. The next week Maria returned and said she understood why her body had not been responding to the massage. She was involved in a friendship with someone who was repeatedly demanding and dismissive of her needs. She knew this, yet still continued the friendship. Maria started to pay attention to her body and realized that her pelvic tension increased noticeably whenever they made plans or even talked on the phone.

Over the next several months, Maria came for periodic pelvic tune-ups. When she was able to honor herself and maintain her personal boundaries, her pelvic tension decreased significantly, but each time she ignored her instinct to keep her distance from this relationship, she felt an immediate change in her pelvic muscles. Maria recognized a trend of self-denial in several of her relationships that she wanted to change. A woman's body will always reveal the truth of her outer life, and she must choose to honor or dishonor herself by accepting or denying this truth.

As a woman, your body is naturally receptive. However, the pelvic bowl is your sacred space, and you can choose what you receive into your body and your life. Be clear about what you receive and decide whether or not it is beneficial to release the tension held in your left pelvic bowl.

## Posterior-Quadrant Pelvic Tension: Where Is Your Support?
Tension in the lower pelvis often relates to support issues. The posterior pelvic quadrant lies directly in front of the sacrum, and together they provide key structural support for your pelvic bowl. Reflections regarding posterior-quadrant pelvic tension include:

What are you holding in the tension of your posterior pelvis?
What is support to you? How do you want to be supported
in your life?
What other types of support would you like to create for
yourself? Can you receive this support?

### Women's Stories: Building a Base of Support

Lena came to see me for postpartum pelvic work six months
after the birth of her son. At three months postpartum, she
had reconstructive surgery in her posterior pelvic musculature
to repair the significant tear she sustained during labor. She
was a courageous woman, one whose journey defines the
meaning of building a base of support both in the pelvis and
one's personal life.

Lena's husband had unexpectedly filed for divorce two
weeks before the birth of their child, leaving her a single mother,
and she went into labor feeling completely alone and unsup-
ported. Lena said that she was hardly surprised by the tear in her
pelvic muscles because she was extremely tense during birth.

She made it through her son's birth and the transition to
motherhood by taking one step at a time. She had pelvic surgery and then pelvic care to "put her body back together."
Lena had a solid network of friends and a self-described
"stubborn streak" that came in handy for rebuilding her support system.

I have had several clients who have weathered stress or
separations with their partners near childbirth, all of whom
have come to me for treatment to address tears in their posterior pelvic quadrant. When a woman does not feel supported
in her external life, whether because of scarcity or a sense of
being alone, she holds this tension in her posterior pelvic muscles in an attempt to create internal support. Areas of muscular

tension are the most susceptible to general injury, tearing with childbirth, or diminished vitality because a tense muscle loses the suppleness that supports its dynamic functioning.

Your support system can be found in many ways: the solace of nature, a thoughtful act, a place to retreat, the loving presence of a friend or partner, a new way to express yourself, the ability to release an old pattern, a particular mode of self-care, a satisfying creative outlet or career direction, and the helper spirits or ancestors who respond to ritual and prayer—whatever you need in the present moment. Healthy support structures enhance your life by encouraging the expression of your true self. Cultivate external structures that meet your current needs for support, and then allow yourself to rest fully into that support, to reduce the demands on your posterior pelvic bowl.

## Right-Quadrant Pelvic Tension: Where Are You Bold?

Tension held in the right quadrant of the pelvic muscles often relates to issues of stepping out into the world because this quadrant and the right ovary are typically associated with a woman's external creations. Reflections regarding right-quadrant pelvic tension include:

What are you holding in the tension of your right pelvis?
What are you presently creating in the outer world?
What else does your feminine spirit desire to create?

### Women's Stories: Finding Her Success

Jennifer sought treatment to increase her pelvic stability and to resolve a chronic weakness in her right pelvis. She had difficulty engaging the right side of her pelvic muscles and experienced multiple points of tenderness in this region. The painful spots decreased with vaginal massage, allowing her to actively tighten these muscles during a pelvic exercise.

Jennifer returned three weeks later, after trying the self-massage and pelvic mapping at home several times. She noticed that each time she checked herself, the muscles on the right side were painful and tense. They would relax with the pelvic massage, then tighten again the next day.

I asked Jennifer to identify sources of stress in her daily life. She replied that her most significant cause of stress was related to self-esteem. Jennifer thought other people could do whatever they set out to accomplish, but she never allowed herself this same possibility. I told her to imagine a situation that created stress for her because of this lack of faith in herself. While she thought of herself at work, where she questioned her level of success, the right quadrant of her pelvic muscles became extremely tense. Though she received continuous positive feedback on her job performance, she often discounted this praise. Jennifer found herself plagued with self-doubt due to her strong inner critic that resisted any personal sense of achievement.

Jennifer was surprised by the direct impact that her stress around self-worth played in her body and wanted to change her self-concept to relieve this tension in her core. I invited her to picture herself doing an activity that gave her confidence, and she imagined swimming, having been an accomplished swimmer and past member of several swim teams. As she did so, her right pelvic tension completely released.

Her body wisdom conveyed to her the consequences of doubting her own capacity. By denying herself or her ability, Jennifer restricted the vast potential of her spirit. The impact of this conflict was evident in the repeated tension she found in her core muscles.

By visualizing herself in an empowering activity, Jennifer restored the energetic and physical sense of empowerment in her root. Following the direction of her body, she joined a gym and returned to swimming as a regular activity. While moving with grace in the water, she pondered taking this inner ease with her to the office. The next time she received praise in her job, she observed her tendency to tighten her body and consciously imagined herself flowing with the water instead. She smiled and accepted the praise, changing her ability to receive validation and embody her potential. By remembering a sense of confidence in her body, Jennifer developed an internal framework for self-confidence as well.

When a woman believes in herself, from her very core, she will find success time and again. Believe in the gifts that you bring to the world and choose what empowers you as a woman to lighten the load on the right side of your pelvic bowl.

## Revitalize Your Pelvic Muscles

The key to vaginal vitality is to actively engage your pelvic muscles in each quadrant. Once your pelvic muscles are moving and accessing their full range, they can be further revitalized. Holding a sustained squat position (such as while working in the garden) is a dynamic way to increase the stamina of your pelvic muscles, while using internal massage to release tension and then simply doing your daily exercise routine (whether walking, working out at the gym, or practicing the stance poses of yoga) will further ensure a robust pelvic floor. Be creative in working with your pelvic bowl and strengthening your core connection.

### Exercise: Affirming Your Core Radiance

This is a standing exercise to energize the blood and chi of your pelvic bowl. Use it to clear stagnation after prolonged sitting, as part of your self-care routine, or anytime you desire to affirm your core radiance.

1. Engage your pelvic floor. Squeeze your root muscles and feel them engage, acknowledging your vibrant center. Then release your pelvic muscles, letting go of anything that does not reflect your dynamic nature. Repeat five times, consciously nourishing your body and affirming a positive connection with your root.

2. Perform hip circles. Stand with your feet together and move your hips in a circle, as if tracing an imaginary hula hoop. Circle five times one way, then five times the other way. Now repeat with your feet spread hip-width apart and widen your circles. Try to make smooth, wide circles and notice that you are circling your body in your own energy field, circulating the energy as you do so.

3. Shake and tap. Shake out your pelvis by bending at the knees in a rapid up and down motion and tap all around your pelvic bowl with your hands. Move your pelvis and feel the vibration down through your legs and feet to the earth. Like slapping or shaking the dust out of a rug, you are revitalizing the blood and energy flow in your pelvic bowl.

4. Align your heart and bowl. Place one hand over your heart and the other hand over the front of your pelvic bowl, feeling the connection between these two places. It is said that a woman has two hearts because of the heart-like energy of the womb. Let these two places align with one another, in silence or with a blessing such as: *I am a divine creation of the universe.*

5. Bring in light energy. Gather the rainbow hues of light energy by stretching your arms out as far as they will reach, and then imagine sweeping this energy toward your body. Repeat this motion in all directions around your body. The radiant energy

of the universe comes to us more readily when we call from the center of our being.

New body patterns are established by working with the body over time. To change a core body pattern requires touch (to initiate change in the physical pattern), breath (to change the energy flow), movement (to integrate the pattern), and repetition (to reinforce the new pattern). By doing vaginal massage and directing breath toward the pelvic bowl, you will begin to change your core patterns. By repeating your root care over time, the new, more beneficial patterns will be integrated and sustained. This process of reshaping your pelvic bowl and increasing your creative energy flow can be assisted by repeating mantras (intentions or beliefs repeated to help create new energy patterns):

> *My root is a vibrant place.*
> *I create what I want.*
> *I am a radiant woman.*
> *I love my female form.*

Another way to access your core vitality is to address the wants and needs reflected in your pelvic space. Ponder your pelvic tensions and strengths to receive the guidance they contain for you.

### Exercise: Reflecting on Your Pelvic Space

1. Bring your attention to your pelvic space and visualize what you are presently creating in your life.

2. Ask your root what nourishment you need and what external structures will bring more support.

3. You have all the tools in your pelvic space to create what you want, and you can seek your sources of strength as sustenance

on this journey. Look to your sources of tension to address any unacknowledged needs.

4. Let in the grace of spirit, and your center will reflect the true capacity of your feminine nature.

### Your Pelvic Self-Care Tools

Practice these self-care tools as part of your daily routine, particularly in response to an increase in stress, an intensely emotional experience, or any significant pelvic event. Take care of your root and discover a new relationship with the tremendous resource that is your female body, using it as a guide and gauge for your overall well-being.

> **Shower Check:** In your morning shower, place a finger in your vagina to quickly gauge your current level of pelvic health or imbalance. Just touching your perineum is grounding, bringing your energy down to an internal and quieter place. Notice the state of your pelvic muscles. Are they tense and holding excess stress, or are they supple and relaxed? Are you holding tension for any unmet needs? If so, how can you provide for yourself and release this pelvic tension? Becoming familiar with your root on a regular basis is essential for your self-care. It will assist you in receiving your root wisdom as it arises.

> **Pelvic Bowl Meditation:** Take a moment to meditate on your pelvic bowl. What kind of feelings or energy are you holding here? Is this what you want to cultivate in your life? Your female body has the power to create whatever you hold in your center. Reaffirm your presence in your own creative core by choosing what to keep in your bowl.

**Vaginal Massage:** Utilize your internal massage techniques to restore your pelvic presence and release chronic pelvic muscle tension. Do a session of vaginal massage after discovering a pelvic imbalance or when simply feeling out of sorts. As you touch internally, ask your body what is held in each place of tension. Invite your body to release whatever it is ready to let go of. Make love with the intention of receiving an internal massage from your partner.

**Expand Awareness with Pelvic Mapping:** To receive the wisdom of your core feminine place, pay attention to the response of your pelvic space in the midst of everyday events. Combine your daily awareness with mapping your pelvic floor, noticing the patterns of tension that result from external events. Learn to read your pelvic muscles like a map and to discover what is needed to restore your creative flow.

**Receive Regular Pelvic Care:** Have pelvic work done periodically as part of your women's healthcare routine (and particularly after any pelvic trauma or stressful life event) by a therapist trained in Holistic Pelvic Care or a women's health physical therapist who specializes in treating the pelvic floor with vaginal bodywork. Maya Abdominal Massage (the Arvigo Techniques) is a beautiful bodywork practice that cultivates uterine and pelvic alignment. Developed by Rosita Arvigo, based on her study with Don Elijio Panti, a traditional Maya healer from Belize, these techniques have attracted a growing national and global network of practitioners. Restoring pelvic balance on a regular basis and preventively addressing pelvic wounds will serve your long-term health, wellness, and creative vitality as a woman.

**Laugh, Sing, and Nourish Yourself:** The muscles of the mouth and pelvis are related to one another. They are connected physiologically and also in their purpose. The pelvic space relates to your feminine creativity, a form of your personal expression. The mouth and jaw are also involved in your self-expression. Because of these connections, relaxing the jaw muscles decreases pelvic tension. Opening your expression through laughter, song, and other nurturing activities restores your feminine spirit and reenergizes your root.

I think the root has a sense of humor. My work has provided me with many occasions for laughter. When one of my sons was about three, we were shopping at our neighborhood store, buying groceries for our home and supplies for my office. As the checker rang up the rubber gloves that I was purchasing for work, my son announced proudly, "My mama works with vaginas!" I smiled at her surprised expression. After the birth of my third son, I received a package in the mail from a colleague. Assuming it was a baby gift, I opened it while rocking the baby and chatting with my mother-in-law. Peeling off the paper I found a large velvet vagina puppet (made, of course, in San Francisco). My mother-in-law raised her eyebrows and said, "Hmm." The root says, *Lighten up and laugh.*

*May you laugh and live from your root.*

# THREE

# Embodying Your Womanhood

*The feminine is our access point to the greater realm of spirit, yet most of our concepts of the feminine are restrictive and inaccurate portrayals of this profound way of being. As if looking at a vast landscape through a pinhole, we are missing the beauty that is right next to us. This chapter invites the exploration and expansion of the conceptual feminine to begin a relationship with this mystery present within our bodies and lives.*

*B*irthing my own children and working with women, I have seen that the root of the female body is a place for being with spirit, a holy center where babies and other creative seeds are planted. These womb seeds are tended by the wild feminine, a presence as old and untamed as the wind.

Women long to connect with this ancient wild feminine energy and to tap into its creative potential, yet most of our creations are shaped by the demands of the outer world rather than by the inner rhythm of our bodies. Like a land no longer inhabited, the womb lies forgotten. Only when a woman seeks to become pregnant will she plant her creative seeds with urgency. After the birth of her baby, she will likely forget her womb just when she needs it for mothering. If a woman does not carry a child, she may never venture into this fertile place within her. Whether or not a woman gives birth, her female body houses her feminine creative energy. A woman must reclaim the feminine terrain of her body to access her full creative range.

When feminism liberated women from their domestic roles, no one was left to tend the home fire, this sacred space where the inner life is nurtured and sustained. The root of the female body embodies the energy of the home and so mourns this loss. No longer tied to the home and the land, our lives contain more choice and greater freedom. Still, our female bodies move in sync with the natural rhythms and ancient roles that once defined our sense of place. In many walks of life, new modes of integrating home and work are essential, and the root has valuable answers to help harmonize the inner and outer in soulful and satisfying ways. We can draw upon the root to bring in the energy required to shape our modern lives in ways that honor our feminine and inherently creative selves.

## Redefine Your Feminine Identity

I have yet to see a woman come into my practice who already fully embodies the root of her female body. When a woman is in tune with her core, she has a robust energetic presence in the pelvic bowl, which she carries into her daily life, and she knows how to maintain that. This serves her both in challenging situations, such as during a conflict or when external circumstances are not meeting her expectations, and in moments of pleasure to celebrate her joy. When fully embodying her root, a woman can access her core energy to heal her feminine wounds. She can release self-limiting patterns and engage her potential.

To change any core pattern, a woman can work with the creative and feminine energy that is meant to flow in her body.

Though the women I see for pelvic care have modern beliefs about their roles in contemporary society and feel themselves to be empowered, inwardly their bodies register discomfort with many aspects of their femininity. This is the result of feminine wounding and restrictive female identities. Women often reject their feminine nature in response to the limitations imposed upon them by the outside world and, in doing so, limit their access to feminine energy.

There is an alternative. Rather than living with only a fraction of her identity, a woman can challenge the gender constructs that restrict it. When a woman begins to examine the roles and choices she associates with femininity, she can begin to change them. Each woman has the right and the desire to express the feminine in her own unique way: a woman's creative potential depends upon her ability to take advantage of this freedom. In forging a direct relationship with the feminine, a woman consciously reclaims and cultivates her own creative ground.

## A Personal Meaning of the Feminine

The first step in redefining your feminine identity is to assess what the feminine means to you. Use the following exercise to assist you in this process.

### Exercise: Assessing Your Meaning of the Feminine

Begin with a piece of paper and pen.

1. List all the things that you associate with being a woman.

2. List all the things that you associate with being feminine.

3. Reflect on the similarities and differences between these two lists.

Questions for reflection:

Did you tend to list roles, issues, adjectives, or parts of the body?

What does that imply about your view of womanhood and the feminine?

How are your lists similar? How are they different?

Is there anything listed that you want to change for yourself?

What do you need to support this change?

Is there anything you desire to add for yourself?

What is needed to bring this feminine aspect into your life?

When I did the exercise myself, I associated being a woman primarily with body-based terms: vagina, birth, breasts, blood. I also listed a few negative words (*disrespected* and *unheard*) as well as the role of mother. Although the word *mother* had positive connotations for me, it is perhaps not a coincidence, given the Western cultural tendency to marginalize motherhood, that it was on the same list as the negative qualities I expressed in relation to womanhood. Words came slowly as I pondered associations with *woman*, yet I found that *woman*, rather than *feminine*, was the term I primarily identified with. Though I did not connect directly to the word *feminine*, my list of associations flowed freely: beautiful, open, sensual, receptive, expressive, playful. It surprises me that no negative terms came to mind in my exploration of *feminine*. In fact, I noticed that the related words were more descriptive and less restrictive than my associations with *woman*.

As I began to interpret the results of this exercise, I realized that I had lived and identified primarily with myself as *woman*. The limitations I felt, expressed on my first list, were primarily based on external definitions of womanhood I had encountered or on my experiences as a woman. However, meditating on the word *feminine* spoke to something in me that had remained untouched. I began to feel that if I could perceive the feminine within my female body, I would find the expansive nature of my spirit.

Another woman may uncover a similar relationship, or her associations may be completely different, depending on her experiences in her female body and on her personal relationship to the feminine. The goal of this exercise is to discover what each of us needs to create and embody our own expression of femininity.

## Daughters and Sons: The Pink Boots

I was glad to be a girl. I liked my body and other aspects of girlhood, and I never once wanted to be a boy. Imagine my surprise at the relief I felt, years later, when I looked at my first newborn babe and saw that he was a son.

By the time I was pregnant a second time, I was well aware of my hesitation to have a daughter. These feelings seemed foreign. How could I, who loved the company of women, feel uneasy at the thought of a daughter? It seemed my notions of female gender equality had missed their mark somewhere along the way.

My comfort with sons and discomfort with daughters have to do with my ambivalence about certain aspects of womanhood. Not expecting to encounter this reaction in myself, I searched for its origin. I was raised in a religion that spoke of God—and those in closest relationship to God—as male. In school, lesson upon lesson reinforced the absence of women in history, politics, and all things worthy of study.

As I sifted through my past, I found no single explanation for my response to mothering a girl. However, I realized that in many subtle ways I had shed trappings of femininity, like softness and vulnerability or even wearing skirts, that seemed to interfere with the perception of myself as strong or capable.

In becoming a woman, I had repeatedly parted ways with my feminine nature. Burdened by the restrictive definitions of feminine beauty, I abandoned them and, in doing so, lost touch with my own love of beauty. Learning that tenderness can be taken advantage of, I steeled myself, accepting little to no help and turning over my feminine ability to receive. In my early years of school, my inner feminine longed to take art and philosophy classes but my focus was oriented toward achievement, and I made choices based on a linear career path that left me feeling empty. These sacrifices were not without a price. My fears about a daughter revealed that I was not entirely happy about these acts of self-betrayal. A daughter would remind me of what I had surrendered. A daughter would also invite me to reclaim what my core self ached for. By mothering a girl, I would traverse lost ground. I was not sure that I felt sufficiently brave.

Ultimately, having sons did not save me from having to confront these issues. Mothering them allowed me to witness the ways that the feminine is stripped from boys. Though the methods may vary, the feminine is discouraged just as detrimentally from both girls and boys. I stepped onto the same lost ground, but I came to it from another direction: the male perspective.

One day, I was shopping in a children's clothing store filled with organic clothing, wooden blocks, and other natural materials indicative of a thoughtful proprietor. My eldest son, then three years old, saw a collection of rain boots for sale. He picked out a pair of pink ones with cats on them.

"Mama, can I have these boots?" he asked.

Before I could answer, the owner of the store swept them from his hands. "These aren't your size. I'll just put them back for you." Then she winked at me and whispered, "I know you don't want him wearing pink boots. I'll pretend we're out of this color."

I answered her out loud, so my son could hear, "Actually, it's okay with me if he has pink boots. I believe those are his size." My son stepped up to the woman, took the boots back, and placed them solidly into the paper bag holding our other purchases. He touched my leg and eyed the store owner warily.

When we were in our car, I said to my son, "You picked out some wild boots, honey." He asked why the store owner had taken them away at first. I explained that most people think of pink as a color for girls only and that other colors, like blue, were considered boys' colors.

He clasped his arms over his chest. "I wear any color I like," he declared.

"That's right, honey," I answered with equal zeal. We were changing the operative code, at least until we got home and my husband, seeing his son's new boots, said, "Why did you let him pick out pink boots?"

When my husband—my proactive, equality-minded, nurturing, modern man of the house—reacted negatively to those boots, I realized that the world would shape my son just as much as I would. After our son went to bed, my husband and I had a long discussion about those pink boots. But we were talking about more than a color; we were delving into gender identity and the wounds that result from the absence of the feminine.

In cultures that are focused on production, where continual output is emphasized rather than natural cycles, the feminine is devalued. This has caused every one of us to disown aspects of our feminine nature. Our children are inadvertently influenced to do the same.

In a natural evolutionary process, that which is deemed unnecessary is eventually left behind. Each member of a given group desires to be productive, that is, to know their value in the presence of others. In order to realize their worth, boys and girls willingly disown the feminine or seemingly unimportant parts of themselves—or risk being devalued. The feminine becomes endangered, and in its place is a gaping hole. Later, each man and woman who forgoes the feminine will yearn for its presence without even remembering what was let go.

I wanted my son to have equal access to color, beauty, and self-expression—in essence, I wanted him to maintain connection with the feminine. My husband wanted to protect this same child from being teased by schooling him in the ways of being a boy and later a man. We were both right. My perspective that rigid gender identities need to be challenged and changed was correct. My husband's view that the culture we live in still operates by gender rules and that we ought to prepare our son to encounter these unspoken boundaries was valid too.

Two years later, after the birth of a second child, my son's pink boots were worn out from days of gardening and digging in our yard. He put them on with ease, unless someone from outside our family was around. In that case, he still wore them but announced, "Pink is not my favorite color."

I guess it was inevitable, the appearance of self-consciousness about the color of his boots. Still, I hope that my sons will find ample room for the expression of the feminine in their lives. Daughters and sons both deserve full access to color and the greater regions of the feminine that it defines.

But restoring the feminine for our children is more complex than giving them equal access to color. What it requires, and where we most often fail, is honesty in the face of our discomfort with the feminine in ourselves. For my sons to retain their connection to the feminine, I went where I was afraid to go with a daughter: to the places where I had abandoned the feminine myself.

I needed courage to revisit my relationship with the feminine, regardless of the gender of my children. And it was not just my own relationship that I have had to address, but the state of the feminine at large. The absence of the feminine and the surprising lack of awareness regarding her absence repeatedly affect my sons in their interactions with others.

Traversing my own lost ground, I remembered why I was glad to be a girl. I learned how to advocate for the feminine in my sons and found a new way of being with boys. I rediscovered pink for myself, as well as other feminine shades of identity and expression that I had rejected long ago in order to avoid the baggage, the *girlie* connotations, they came with. I realized how far I had come when one day, out of the blue, I was glad at the thought of a daughter. I finally loved the girl, the feminine within.

## Creating New Expressions of the Feminine

While working one-on-one with women, I realized the need to explore some of the issues regarding the feminine in a community context. I began teaching classes about the energy system of the female body and the ways that women can use their root energy to renew their feminine expression. In one of my classes, several women were inspired to go further and discover a unique and personal relationship to the feminine.

One woman, a potter, made a vagina bowl. She shaped her clay while pondering her relationship with her body, and she invited other women to gather and create vagina bowls. Each one reflected the essence of the woman who made it. One bowl was inscribed with symbols like a cave; another was carved like a tree. These women went on to make womb bowls, clay ovaries, and masks representing various feminine identities. Another woman was an architect. She thought about the intentional use of space in her designs and the application of these principles for making boundaries and defining the energy held in her body. Another woman had training in martial arts. Based on the discipline and form of her martial arts practice, she pondered ways of reclaiming the more infinite form of her own feminine nature. My own roles as a mother and healer have directed my exploration of the feminine, deepening my awareness for the ancient lines of energy that flow through our bodies and lives.

If every woman recovers the range of the feminine in her own way, we will collectively regain our whole wild feminine landscape. Look to the aspects of your own femininity that desire acknowledgement. Draw upon your areas of expertise. As you begin to acknowledge the feminine in various realms of your life, you will be able to expand your expression in these places. Explore the feminine in your home, work, partnerships, mothering, creative projects, spiritual practice, and any areas in which you desire a direct relationship with the wild feminine.

## Honoring and Dishonoring Your Feminine Self

The next step in understanding your womanhood is to examine where your feminine self is honored or dishonored. The following "I Am Woman" survey will assist your assessment. Take it now to see where you are beginning, and then repeat it along your journey to mark your progress. If you are not sure what a particular question means, take some time to ponder or even freewrite on what you think it might mean to you. There is no right or wrong way to honor yourself as a woman. These questions are designed to help you discover the desires of your feminine self.

### Exercise: I Am Woman Survey

Answer the following questions according to this range of responses, placing the respective number next to each statement:

Never (-2)        Unsure (-1)
I'd like to (0)     Sometimes (1)
Definitely (2)

_____ I celebrate my femininity.
_____ I have a regular creative practice.
_____ I make time to enjoy my creations.
_____ I nourish my female body.
_____ I follow my own inherent rhythms.
_____ I access my root wisdom.
_____ I routinely utilize my tools for holistic pelvic self-care
to restore balance in my core.

_____ I acknowledge my feminine wounds and claim my feminine gifts.

_____ I think of my pelvis as sacred space.

_____ I consciously embrace my lineage and pay attention to what I am passing on.

_____ I challenge cultural and family myths regarding femininity.

_____ I embody my own unique expression of the feminine.

_____ I hold my ground and advocate for my needs as a woman.

_____ I embrace my full feminine radiance.

_____ Total Score

Now tally up your score and assess how well you honor yourself as a woman. The maximum score is 28, though the goal is not necessarily achieving a certain number, but rather accomplishing an internal sense of where and how you might enhance your ability to honor your feminine self. For any statements that received a score of 0 or below, ask yourself how you would like to be honored or newly engaged in this aspect of your femininity.

## Find Your Root Voice

For a woman to make her own relationship with the feminine, she must find her root voice. This is the clear and honest voice of a woman's core feminine self. When she focuses her attention on the root of her body, a woman will often hear this voice that reflects her maternal and creative wisdom. This inner root voice will always acknowledge the places a woman has relinquished her power, forgotten her creative dreams, or tends to forgo her own well-being.

Women are often surprised by the personality, even wit, that comes through when they listen to the root. Eve Ensler captures the nature of the root voice in her play *The Vagina Monologues*,

which she wrote after interviewing hundreds of women about their
vaginas. Every woman's root voice is unique. One voice will sing
sweetly, *You are so right*, and another will yell loudly, *Not that way*.
Depending on the situation a woman is responding to, every root
tone has its purpose. Exploring the various tones of the root voice
allows a woman to find aspects of her feminine self that desire to be
heard and developed.

### Women's Stories: Discovering a New Voice

Marianne sought pelvic care to address her muscular imbalances. As her pelvic presence and core musculature became
stronger, she found herself listening to a new voice. By bringing attention to her pelvic area, Marianne found that some of
her bodily needs—such as spending time in her garden—
became a priority.

Digging in the dirt, Marianne was more aware of her body.
While tending her garden, she pondered the imbalances in her
life. Marianne typically maintained a busy schedule, ignoring
her physical needs and leaving little time for taking care of
herself. But by heeding the promptings of her body, Marianne
slowed her pace and followed her desire to go outside and
touch the earth. Through her body, Marianne recovered her
physical connection to the ground. A woman's root will
always remind her how to nourish herself, restoring her
natural rhythm and encouraging her to find respite from the
repetitive stress of daily demands.

### Learn to Listen: Internalize Your Value

To be able to listen to her own center, a woman must value herself.
This means that women must attune to themselves first rather than
simply following or pleasing the outer world. With too much
emphasis placed on externalized value, a woman is unable to hear

what lies in her center. Her creations may be attempts to give herself a sense of value. If instead a woman comes from her center, then she knows her inherent value and she brings this value to the world. She creates and lives not from a void, but from the abundant beauty that arises from her core.

To hear the voice of your root, begin to find your center. Your center means the center of your body but also the core areas of creative joy in your life. Begin this practice by guiding your attention from your head down to your pelvis. Bring your breath and your focus to the base of your pelvic bowl. Take a moment to listen. What is your root saying to you? Where is your creative joy?

Now visualize a particular situation that challenges you in your life. Respond first with your head voice and then with your root voice. Do you sense the difference? Your head voice will say things like: *I wonder what they think about what I am doing* or *I should do this* or *I don't really have a preference.* Your head voice will often compromise your truth, be vague, or trivialize your needs. Your root voice will say: *This is what I know* or *my strength is here* or *I'll take that one.* Your root voice will be honest, direct, creative, and serve your best interest. Let her guide you.

### Exercise: Finding Your Root Voice

1. Reflect upon a situation in which you felt unsure in some way. Review the situation in your mind and try to think it through.

2. Thinking always involves your head voice. Now bring your awareness down to your pelvic space and feel your response. This deep inner knowing is the voice of your root, or feminine intuition.

3. Notice the difference in the assuredness and potential outcome of feeling rather than thinking through your response.

Generally, you will find that your feminine spirit does not feel compromised when speaking from this powerful place.

4. Though it may be awkward initially, with practice you will find your root voice with ease. Ponder what is needed to access your root voice on a regular basis.

## Give Voice to Your Root

Your root voice speaks from your deepest feminine self. Whenever you feel lost, come back here to listen. She is strong. She is vital. She is the expression of your authentic woman.

By acknowledging the full range of emotions that accompanies your experience of womanhood, you give voice to your root. You may ask: *What do emotions have to do with my pelvic health?* Emotions are a form of expression, and unexpressed emotions are often held within the core of the body. They become obstacles to energy flow and create physical tension, particularly in your lower belly, vagina, and pelvic muscles. As a result, your root becomes a container for the energy of these unexpressed emotions. Acknowledging buried feelings and releasing the contained energy is essential for your vital energy flow and the clarity of your root voice. On this journey to recover your wild femininity, every emotion encountered in your root has a purpose in recovering your root expression.

Notice the emotions you tend to express or suppress. Use the following exercise to assist you in this process.

### *Exercise: Emotional Assessment*

Finish the following statements:

1. The primary emotion associated with my experience as a woman is ...

2. I think I feel this way because ...

3. I often find myself feeling ...

4. I rarely feel ...

5. I allow myself to express ...

6. I suppress the emotional state of ...

7. The women in my family often feel/felt ...

8. The men in my family primarily express/expressed ...

9. Others would describe my typical emotional state as ...

Listening to the range of expression in the root voice, I have come to appreciate the powerful movement of energy through a woman's body as she accesses a previously buried emotion. You can work with an emotion as it arises or examine certain emotional patterns of expression or suppression. Emotional patterns often provide clues about where core energy is blocked and held in or flowing unsustainably. Suppressing emotions takes a great amount of energy and limits access to joy as well. The ability to feel and express emotions is essential to live with passion.

Acknowledging feelings held in the core allows for their expression. The movement of this emotional energy often leads to a healing action. For example, anger can bring forward latent powers; sadness invites a reconnection with aspects of spirit; grief strips away old forms of being and prepares for the way ahead.

Strong feelings arise in the process of recovering the range of the wild feminine. The pain carried in your body often echoes genera- tions of loss, and it takes time to move through the layers of feelings held in your pelvic bowl. The emotions encountered during this process may be intimidating, but each signifies the potential to reclaim another piece of feminine ground. (I have provided additional stories and information about specific emotions and their purpose in chapters 3 through 7 for further exploration.)

The root voice speaks with the rich variety of feminine expression. Open any places of constriction and see what begins to flow. Reflections on your emotions include:

What is the predominant essence of your root voice?

How does this tone change as you encounter different experiences?

What aspects of your root voice remain unheard or only occasionally surface?

## Work with Your Emotional Energy

Women are emotional by nature. Accessing the feminine allows us to tap directly into the powerful emotional currents that give rise to passion and creative energy. As we open ourselves to the feminine, initially we can feel overwhelmed by some of the emotional storms that we encounter. These feelings are important; they teach us about ourselves—our needs and our desires. By learning to work with the emotional energies, we can receive guidance for healing and enhancing our creative flow. However, we need to move the emotional energy rather than simply reacting with a habitual pattern. Working at the edge between energy flow and physical body, we can engage and change core patterns to benefit our well-being. Use the following exercise to expand your potential when encountering a surge of emotions.

### Exercise: Working with Emotional Energy

1. Ask yourself: How am I feeling?

2. Ask: Where do I feel this in my body?

3. Do you have a sense of balance and a root connection in your pelvic bowl right now?

4. If not, feel the connection between the base of the pelvic bowl and the earth. Choose a pelvic exercise to clarify and balance the pelvic energy (sitting on the ground is helpful).

5. Once you feel a grounded and balanced pelvic connection, ask the following questions:

   • Is there something I need to be aware of or heal for myself? Take note of what you are learning and what this emotion is conveying to you.
   • What type of care do I need in the present moment? Taking care of yourself further assists your body in clearing the emotional energy and healing the energetic layers.
   • What do I want? This question harnesses the potential of your creative power.

6. Bring your awareness back to your body again. Become aware of the beauty of the present moment. Notice the quality of light, your breath, and the sensations of your body, and concentrate your attention on what is good. Positive thoughts support alignment of your own energy center; continue to hold your desired intention.

## The Vagina Timeline

The next step after locating your root voice is to acknowledge the path you have traveled as a woman. Reflect on your life and womanhood, thinking about what defines your femininity. Identify where you have been wounded in body or spirit. Ponder your feminine strengths and desires. Notice the places of disconnection from your vagina, womb, or feminine self.

I suggest creating a vaginal timeline, a variation of an exercise from Clarissa Pinkola Estes's book *Women Who Run with the Wolves*, to help you acknowledge the experiences that have shaped you as a woman. Just as roadside crosses mark remembrances of the dead, Estes suggests making a timeline with crosses acknowledging the descansos, or "resting places," in one's own life.

### *Exercise: Making a Vagina Timeline*

1. Begin by drawing a long line to represent the time from your conception to your present age. Divide your age in half and write this number at the center point of your timeline. Divide each side of the timeline into sections, one for each year of your life.

2. Identify events associated with your female body or femininity that moved or changed you in some way. Listen to your root voice for any other experiences that come to mind. Record them on your timeline with a symbol of your choice that reflects your womanhood. Ponder the influence of these events in the formation of your feminine identity and your creative life.

### Healing and the Potential of Being Witnessed

As you explore the root of your female body, you will encounter wounds, places of grief and pain associated with your body or femininity that you tend to avoid. However, the best way to recover lost feminine ground is to examine these wounds. By attending to them and remembering the losses they mark, you are bearing witness.

One of the most challenging aspects of wounds associated with the most intimate place in the female body is the silence, secrecy, shame, or isolation that tends to trap energy. The process of witnessing the truth of these wounds, of acknowledging the pain, of being seen and heard by another person, allows it to begin to move.

Witnessing can take place in private, with each woman testifying to the truth of her journey (for example, in the making of a vagina timeline). A close friend or teacher can witness as you share an experience. Witnessing can also be done in a group context, with a ritual or specified gathering.

When a wound is witnessed, its energy begins to change. Instead of remaining held in the energy field of the body, it becomes observable and movable. You can interact with it and shape it, dissipating its power or held energy. Energy previously spent to contain the wound is now available for use in another, more conscious way.

The wounds related to your womanhood define you only if they prevent you from owning and accessing the vibrant energy of your core. You cannot change what has happened to you, but you can change the way it impacts the root of your body. Your pelvic energy is rich and radiant. By taking care of your root on a daily basis and spending time in its warmth, you will be defined by this radiance more and more.

## Shame: Reclaim Your Ground

The primary emotion blocking women from their root power is shame. Disrespect for the feminine nature has led both women and men to carry a sense of shame about their own feminine aspects. The female body is shamed. Shame is unpleasant, and we naturally separate ourselves from anything we consider shameful. When a woman associates her womanhood with shame, she becomes separated from essential parts of her vital self and loses vast regions of her feminine ground.

When I began my women's health practice, I sensed inexplicable feelings of sadness or intangible loss during pelvic care sessions.

There was a well of emotion and knowledge held in the pelvic space that I was aware of at a deeper level. As I began to honor each woman's pelvic wisdom and potential in her own healing process, I noticed that the sense of sadness dissipated. In acknowledging the root wisdom, a prior loss was healed. Ultimately, this observation caused me to change my work practices.

Instead of emphasizing the myriad pelvic problems a woman can experience and inadvertently adding to the shame she feels about her body, I now speak about the strength and beauty of the pelvic space. I have learned to listen to the wisdom of each woman's body. My priority is teaching prevention and self-care tools in order to empower a woman to heal her own wounds and to restore her own pelvic balance. When a woman has experienced rape or other violations, I assist her in reclaiming her personal power by teaching her to develop a strong pelvic presence. I acknowledge the emotions that may arise with bodywork in the pelvic space and talk about shame directly, so women know what to expect. With every word and action, I strive to work from a place of deep respect for my clients and for the creative resources of their female bodies.

## Women's Stories: Reclaiming Her Space

Rita was interested in pelvic floor work to reconnect with her body. As we began, she found that vaginal massage and pelvic exercises brought up emotions she had difficulty identifying. I suggested that she simply let the energy of these feelings move without trying to understand them. As she tried to find her bearings, I felt Rita's ambivalence about her pelvic space. When I am sitting with a client, my words are always guided by the woman's relationship to her body. Rita told me that focusing on her root made her aware of an almost hatred-like aversion toward her lower body. I shared my perspective that hatred and other aversions are often related to the energy of shame. At their base, emotions are just a concentrated form of energy. The energy of shame can be released from the body, allowing a woman to reclaim this fertile place.

Rita breathed a heavy sigh and poured out her story. She was emotionally abused and neglected as a girl, and she later sought connection with others through her sexuality. As a young woman, she had sex with partners who were often disrespectful to her, and one of these relationships resulted in a pregnancy. Young and single, she felt that abortion was her only option. Telling no one, she went alone to a clinic. Rita bled for days afterward; the silence of her womb was deafening, and finally she learned to ignore this part of her body altogether.

The shame that Rita carried about these painful events discouraged her from connecting with her root. And though a woman may make a decision that feels right to her, still there can be a burden of pain. I have seen the energy pattern of shame in the pelvis of every woman I have worked with. Though each woman has her own reasons for holding shame, it universally restricts a woman's feminine nature. Shame is often held in a place where a woman's energy has been profoundly disrupted and her spirit abandons this ground. Shame serves as a marker for these losses. Grieving with acknowledgment, compassion, ritual, the support of bodywork or counseling, and attention to her center will help to ease these burdens.

Even as Rita shared her story, the energy of her womb changed. If a woman maintains an awareness of this energetic presence in her root, even as shame arises, the energy of shame will clear and she will heal the split in herself that shame has caused for so long. Clearing shame from the pelvic bowl is like letting in light and fresh air to a closed room.

Shame tends to isolate a woman, making her feel as if she is alone in her experience. During our session, my discussion of the universal aspects of shame gave Rita courage. She focused attention on her pelvic bowl, even though it required witnessing a tremendous outpouring of shame and grief. After several minutes of focused breathing, bringing her awareness back into her womb, Rita's feminine energy began to flow again. The sense of shame dissipated, the grief moved, and Rita felt warmth flooding her pelvic space. Returning to the root of her body, Rita found her whole sense of self expanded. To maintain this sense of healing may require more personal work for Rita, but each piece of work will strengthen her presence in the core. As each of us clears the shame and other burdens from our female body, we too can recover our lost feminine ground.

## The Root Voice of Shame: Unrealized Potential

Any shame held in the female body blocks a woman's natural state of wholeness. Female shame—or shame associated with the vagina, womb, or feminine self—limits a woman's ability to inhabit her feminine nature. To avoid this shame, women naturally separate from their femininity and female body. When she disassociates from the feminine within herself, a woman also limits her radiance and ability to protect her feminine ground, both of which require a strong presence in the pelvic bowl.

Every woman has patterns of shame—even just from society's influence of how femininity is allowed to be experienced—in regard to her body. When shame arises while working on the pelvic bowl, I have seen how it immediately stops the flow of a woman's creative energy. I have also learned that shame patterns dissipate with an honoring presence. If a woman encounters a place of shame and then focuses on honoring herself rather than the shame, then the negativity clears and she recovers the full radiance of her creative energies in that same place.

Though honoring yourself in the presence of shame is a simple practice, it requires a conscious effort. When you meet your root voice of shame, the typical first response is to move in the opposite direction. This voice may say: *Honor my vagina? But it's dirty* or *Ugh, not my time of the month again—what a curse.* Shame associated with the pelvic space interferes with caring for this part of your body. Think about how you feel during a pelvic exam. Women who come to me for pelvic work usually do so because they are experiencing symptoms that motivate them to seek help, not because they love their vaginas and want to take care of them.

Shame regarding the female pelvis also discourages healthcare professionals from becoming pelvic care providers, as I discovered when a women's health position opened at the hospital where I had worked. In a staff of twenty-plus therapists, most of them women, not a single other practitioner was interested in training for this position. I saw it as a unique opportunity, having no idea what a wonderful path it would lead me to.

As I began to work with women, I learned a lot about the relationship between women and the root of their bodies. I found that most women were totally or partially disconnected from this place. In fact, none of the women I saw as clients were accessing their root wisdom. Who could know there was such rich potential in the root of the female body?

I found that women were often embarrassed about anything associated with caring for the pelvic space. This was hardly surprising. Women are inundated with advertisements for products designed to help them change their bodies and with powerful messages focusing on the mess—rather than the power—associated with a woman's menstrual cycle. These messages conspire to teach girls and women that their vaginas are dirty and shameful. Other sources of shame arise from early impressions in children when they receive negative messages about the body or bodily functions. Women also learn to carry shame about femininity in general: sources of this shame include self-image, body shape, changes in the body, changes arising from birthing a child, challenges with fertility, the devaluing of the feminine, and the over-sexualization of the root.

Women carry shame from pelvic traumas resulting in self-blame: sexual abuse, rape, abortion, miscarriage, sexually transmitted diseases, and difficult childbirth or birth loss. As my clients fill out the women's health history form at my office, they often express a sense of shame about the particularly painful events related to their womanhood. It is important to acknowledge the negative associations regarding your female body. These are personal, familial, and cultural, but if their energy imprints are unaddressed, they will inhibit you from fully inhabiting your core. In the same manner, clearing these obstacles from the energy of your body will greatly assist you in reclaiming your fertile feminine ground. Clear any shame associated with your female body or feminine nature, restoring a sense of the sacred in its place. This is a direct act to reprogram the internalized messages that otherwise shame and devalue the feminine within yourself.

### Exercise: Clearing Negative Associations from Your Feminine Form

1. Reflections: Take a moment to reflect on any feelings of shame or negative associations regarding femininity or the female body. How have they been dishonored?

2. Ritual: Spend ten minutes freewriting (writing continuously without stopping or editing yourself) every negative word or association that comes to mind regarding your womanhood. When you are finished, fold the paper into a small bundle and burn it (in a safe container). As the paper burns, feel the release in your body from words that restrict your spirit. Now spend ten minutes freewriting about the positive intentions and associations that you would like to hold in your center. Let the words flow freely as you honor your feminine form. When you are finished, place this paper on an altar or plant it in your garden as a blessing for yourself. Ponder this

blessing while nourishing your body and let yourself bask in this loving attention: take a bath, massage yourself with lotion, wear clothing that makes you feel radiant, and so on. Repeat this ritual as needed, replacing negative associations with positive ones until only the positive remain.

*Women's Stories: The Beauty of a Woman's Bleeding Time*

As part of my holistic practice of pelvic care, I have come to appreciate the alternate cycles of holding and releasing in the female body and their inherent purpose in restoring pelvic balance. This awareness shifted my own discontent at the onset of my menstrual bleeding to a sense of welcoming relief. I became grateful for each period, which arrived to clear my pelvic space just when I reached maximum capacity. I have extended this welcoming attitude to my clients.

One week, I worked with six different women bleeding on the same menstrual cycle. It was telling that each woman seemed ashamed by the presence of her blood, apologizing for the "mess." With each woman (and many more since), I shared my perspective that a woman's bleeding correlates to a period of release in her body. Menstruation is a precious gift for our female bodies. Because of our capacity to hold energy, menstruation offers a regular and necessary release of blood and energy. This release clears the womb and pelvic bowl of accumulated energy, releasing what is no longer needed and preparing for the next creative phase. A woman can work with her uterine release (as described in chapter 5) to more effectively clear tension or clarify energy in her pelvic space, even in menopause. The body naturally cleanses and replenishes when we align with our inner cycles.

Each woman appreciated my words. One confided that I was the first person—and certainly the first healthcare practitioner—to tell her that it was good to be bleeding, not an inconvenience or even just a neutral event, but actually a blessing.

## Connect with the Elements of Your Root

Like everything in nature, your body is elemental. Shift your awareness away from any negative body associations and instead remember the basic elemental nature of your body. Find new ways of relating to your core with the following visualization.

### Exercise: Encountering Your Root Elements

Read through the visualization. Then close your eyes and begin. Sense and observe the energy of each organ as you connect with the elements in your root, which may differ as you travel through your bodily and energetic creative cycles.

1. Focus on the center of your pelvic bowl, the uterus. Try to sense the rich and dense place she holds in your pelvis. Because the uterus is one of the strongest muscles in the body, many of the other structures orient themselves around it. It is your core feminine place. The uterus represents the earth element, holding the space to receive the wisdom of your creations. It often reflects an energetic capacity that relates to the seasonal changes of the earth's energy and maintains your creative cycle. Do you honor your feminine wisdom and make space for tending your creations?

2. Now imagine the fluids that flow through your body and your pelvic bowl. The blood that circulates and nourishes your womb as well as the menstrual blood you may shed represent the water element, your emotional feminine self. The lubrication of your vagina and the fluids that are released move in a cyclical manner, like ocean tides. What is your present emotional

state and how is this reflected in your body? Where are you free to let go and express yourself? Where do you feel restricted in this flow?

3. Find a place midway between the top of your pelvic crest and your pubic bone on each side of the front of your pelvis. Just a few inches below this place, on each side, is an ovary. Try to feel the gentle warmth radiating from your ovaries, the fire element in your pelvic space. The fire of the ovaries represents the spark of life or source of all you create. Notice their connection to the central uterus. What is your creative fire presently fueling? Do you receive your own warmth?

4. Broaden your awareness to the whole pelvic bowl and imagine your wild feminine landscape. This is the structure that supports your creative passions. Examine the structures you have built in your life—are they both strong and flexible, able to sustain but also bend as you create? If not, what better ones will serve your creative journey? Notice the edges of your pelvic bowl and the element of air all around you. Make a connection, from within your center, to the energy of spirit. How can you make more room for the lightness of air and receive the fresh inspirations of spirit?

5. Close your visualization and reflect on your observations. Which elements do you most easily respond to? Which elements might enhance your overall creative capacity? Give thanks for your radiant root and your elemental nature.

Incorporating the natural elements into your self-care will further revitalize your root. Encourage the flow of your water element, or emotional nature, by immersing yourself in water, visiting the ocean or another body of water, or finding an outlet for emotional expression. Connect with your air element, or feminine wisdom and spirit, through focused breath, chanting, or observing the sky. Find your fire element, or creative source, through a sauna, hot food, or by meditating on the flames of a fire. Feel your earth element, or feminine ground, by walking barefoot, dancing, or drumming. As you reconnect to your body's elemental nature, you embody your true feminine form.

## Transform Patterns of Pelvic Separation

For a woman to regain her full bodily range, it is essential for her to transform pelvic patterns of separation. For example, many women separate (momentarily dissociate) their awareness from their bodies when undergoing a pelvic exam. Every woman has particular triggers (sex, stress, food, feeling emotionally overwhelmed) that cause her to dissociate from her body and specifically from her pelvic bowl. When dissociation occurs during a stressful event, whether emotional or physical stress, the body feels abandoned and perhaps betrayed. When a woman allows a medical procedure or other pelvic contact to occur without her full presence, her core energy is diminished and her body is less protected.

Women often consent to take on extra loads, compromise themselves, or accept relationship dynamics and other boundary violations that they would avoid if they were fully present in their bodies. If instead a woman can maintain her presence in the root of her body even—especially—when she is challenged, she will receive the grace that comes to her in the moment. Patterns of dissociation can be changed so that a woman is more able to stay grounded in her center, regardless of the situation. She refuses to give up her energetic, physical, or emotional ground and that connection remains intact.

## Practice Pelvic Presence during a Pelvic Exam

Learn how to stay present in the pelvic space by keeping your attention there during your annual pelvic exam. Begin by talking with your body and vagina; let it know what will happen during this procedure and why you are agreeing to it. Prepare yourself to recognize the early signs of disassociation, such as feeling foggy or forgetting where you are. Keep your focus present in the pelvic space during the exam to prevent mentally separating from your body. After the exam, nurture your body by taking a bath or gently rubbing your belly with castor oil and applying a warm cloth. Thank your body for participating in this process for your pelvic health.

When you experience a pelvic examination with full consciousness, you may notice that your pelvis aches afterward. You are less aware of this discomfort when disconnected from your body, but pelvic presence is a tremendous gift to your root. Staying present in the root on a daily basis means being more aware of physical and emotional pain when you are challenged in some way, but it leaves less energetic debris and gives more support. Creating an alliance with your root brings healing to previous violations and offers a new relationship to your womanhood. When you notice shame with your female body or a tendency for pelvic separation, you have the opportunity to transform these patterns. In doing so, you continue to reclaim lost aspects of your wild feminine range. Reflections regarding pelvic presence include:

When do you tend to disassociate from your body?
What potential reconnection lies within your places of separation or shame?
What aspects of your femininity are you proud of?
How can you cultivate and connect with these places of feminine pride?

*Women's Stories: Shame and Feminine Power*

When Joan, a successful businesswoman, came to see me, she was near menopause and experiencing symptoms of mild incontinence. During her internal exam, I found that her pelvic muscles were very tense. Chronic tension inhibits muscle function because it depletes the energy of the cells in the overworking muscle. As I shared my observations about the level of tension in her musculature, Joan replied, with noticeable pain in her voice, that I probably thought she was "uptight." I said that was a word I would never use, but I knew that many powerful women hear such terms from peers, both male and female, who desire to challenge their power.

I acknowledged Joan's pain and my own internal anger at derogatory words that cause women to disown their power. Words like *bitch* imply that empowered women cannot be feminine or sensual, open or soft. Many women who have succeeded in the patriarchal structure of the workplace have denied aspects of their femininity to avoid being considered weak or incompetent.

Joan's pelvic musculature softened with internal bodywork, and perhaps her feminine side softened too in releasing words that no longer served her well-being. Rather than limiting herself with an external label, she could simultaneously celebrate the intensity that led to her accomplished work record and the vast potential within her vital feminine self.

Listen for your own root voice of shame to identify your feminine wounds. If you find a sense of shame associated with any aspect of your female experience including a part of your body, expression, voice, wisdom, or feminine identity, you have the opportunity to reclaim another lost aspect of your feminine range. Because others use shame to diminish your power, it often arises in association with your greatest assets. To reclaim these assets, you must first uncover and witness the shame you have internalized. Witness your shame with the following exercise.

### Exercise: Reclaiming Your Range from Shame

1. Reflection: Take a moment to acknowledge the pain that your female body or feminine spirit has suffered. Think about instances where you split from your womb space or feminine self due to a sense of shame. In regions of shame, ponder what was lost, such as trust, innocence, or a personal trait. Notice whether particular areas of your body are connected with this shame.

2. Ritual: Make a list of your shame on paper by responding to: "I am ashamed of ..." Include as many items as you need. When you are finished, address each item on your list by declaring what you wish to reclaim from each item of shame: "I clear my shame related to ... in order to reclaim the following ... " For example: *I clear my shame related to my female body in order to love and cherish myself; I clear my shame related to my beauty to be able to enjoy my full radiance; I clear my shame related to my miscarriage in order to reclaim a sense of my true fertility; I clear my shame related to my expression to be able to sing out and speak my truth.* Place the paper with your desires for wholeness on an altar or plant it in a garden space. Repeat this exercise whenever your shame arises or blocks you in some way.

Acknowledging your shame will ultimately assist you in restoring your connection to the sacred in your feminine nature and female body. Consciously reclaiming aspects of yourself associated with shame will not make you immune to feeling ashamed, but it will enable you to move the energy of shame. By learning to work with these energies, we receive healing for past wounds and take ownership of our true feminine range. Listen for messages like: *You don't deserve that* or *You shouldn't do that*. Let the root voice of shame be your guide. When shame rises to the surface, you can be certain that you are about to encounter a lost aspect of your feminine range and the potential for its reintegration.

## Renew the Feminine Spirit

As women have struggled with limitations regarding the feminine, they have also found solutions born of these struggles. A prime example is Dr. Christiane Northrup. As an OB/GYN, she had difficulty balancing a career in her male-dominated field with her own feminine perspectives and roles. In her book *Women's Bodies, Women's Wisdom*, she relates the story of how she maintained a heavy workload as a nursing mother, even with a severe breast infection. She needed to rest but feared her peers would think her ineffectual, so she did not allow herself healing time and she lost her ability to produce milk in that breast. This experience motivated her to create her own women's clinic. Dr. Northrup based the mission of this clinic on the way she wanted to practice medicine for her own health as well as for the health of her clients.

Northrup's book describes her practice of women's healthcare, which incorporated a holistic approach that was atypical for mainstream medicine in the early nineties. She published her book in 1994, despite her fear of being mocked by more traditional colleagues. However, *Women's Bodies, Women's Wisdom* was well received and now serves as a textbook in several medical training programs. Northrup provides an uplifting example of a woman bringing change to her field by honoring, rather than denying, her feminine self.

Renewing the feminine spirit means that we, women and men, will bring forth our powers of reception, nurturance, creativity, and intuition—the essence of our feminine selves—into the workplace and our habits of daily living. Then, together, we will be able to work for change in the structures which presently serve monetary objectives rather than human needs.

### Exercise: Inviting the Feminine into Everyday Living

1. Ponder your relationship with the feminine. Do something that invites the dreamy presence of the feminine into the present moment, such as listening to music, gathering a bouquet of flowers, dancing, singing, or wearing something beautiful.

2. Now treat yourself to something that enlivens your body: a tasty meal or a leisurely nap to reinvigorate yourself. Make new and daily connections between your relationship with the feminine and your body. This will remind you that you are free to create and embody your own feminine form.

Each connection that you make between the feminine and a vibrant presence in your body, which you then incorporate into your daily living practices, will shift your associations with the concept of femininity. With each shift, you will embody (physically, energetically, spiritually) more of your own expression of the feminine, infusing every day with your wild feminine energy. Some examples of these practices include:

- Doing pelvic self-care for healing and revitalizing your vagina, uterus, ovaries, and whole pelvic bowl
- Examining pelvic patterns to challenge and redefine inherited expectations of women's roles in society, mothering, partnership, spiritual practice, inner home, and outer work
- Celebrating your female form with loving words, respectful touch, and expressions of your beauty

- Gathering with the vibrant women in your community
- Tending your creative seeds
- Expanding your creativity or sensuality to further reclaim your feminine landscape
- Accessing energetic tools to clear your pelvic space and refocus your creative energy
- Holding your female body as a sacred place to honor the divine aspects of your womanhood
- Listening to your root voice to acknowledge what you hold in your female body and to receive your own feminine wisdom

## The Changing Voice of Female Shame

The shame associated with femininity is often passed through generations. In your pelvic space, you carry messages at a cellular level about what it means to be a woman in your family and your culture. You hold the pain and the potential that is passed on from woman to woman. The rage covering unexpressed creative genius in your grandmother or the mental illness of your great-aunt may be linked to shame, discouraging you from identifying with any traits you share with them.

The gift of each generation is new potential and awareness: an evolution for every woman who pays attention to the changes around her and embraces new modes of being. After working with women from ages twenty to eighty-five, I can see the generational progress in acknowledging women's bodies and feminine selves. Women today have a greater willingness to talk about regions of the body previously buried under mounds of shame. In the process, we are also uncovering and beginning to attend to our various unmet needs. When we acknowledge and nourish our female bodies, we are better able to care for our feminine selves and recognize our feminine desires. Several stages of pelvic self-care are listed below. Where are you on this continuum? Where would you like to be?

1. Unaware of pelvic needs or imbalances, avoids the pelvic region, perhaps seeking pelvic care as recommended by a doctor.

2. Motivated to seek care for symptoms of urine leakage or pelvic imbalance, focused on exercises or external feedback rather than own touch or pelvic self-care.

3. Interested in postpartum or some other aspect of pelvic healing, willing to learn self-care but not necessarily applying these tools.

4. Seeking to connect with her female organs and pelvis for herself, learns and actively applies pelvic self-care tools, aware of the potential and beauty of her pelvic bowl, teaches others about healing and honoring the feminine spirit and how these actions connect to care of the female body.

Identify every remnant of shame associated with your female body in order to fully reclaim your wild feminine. Shame interferes with your ability to honor yourself. Shed this shame and prepare to receive your own sacred femininity.

## Restore Your Sacred Center

Shame effectively maintains a separation between a woman and the root of her body; honoring the root is a potent antidote. One of the most powerful acts a woman can make is to honor her body and her root as sacred. Restoring a sense of the sacred in the pelvic bowl ultimately creates a space that a woman's awareness will joyfully inhabit.

For centuries, organized religions have excluded women from certain aspects of celebrating the divine. They have also taught that a woman's body is unclean. At the same time, earth-based spiritual practices, which honor natural cycles and the female body, were degraded. As a result, many women have subtly or directly separated their female being from their spirituality. They have disowned their inherent connection to spirituality and lost touch with the sacred feminine.

The sacred feminine celebrates the feminine aspects of spirituality. From this perspective, the divine is present in the female body, feminine creativity, sexuality, birth, creative cycles, and motherhood. Recovering an awareness of the sacred within your own womanhood allows you to receive the blessings in these and other uniquely female events. You gain access to your ability to co-create with the divine when you celebrate the sacred feminine in your root.

### Women's Stories: Honoring the Female Body

Maia initially came for bodywork to prepare herself for pregnancy. In addition to restoring her vitality, pelvic awareness exercises helped Maia restore her sacred center. This was a new experience for her; a history of abuse, a past eating disorder, and lingering feelings of shame limited her ability to fully connect with or cherish her body.

As a result of her personal wounds and body disconnect, Maia worried about pregnancy. She both desired and feared the possibility of having a child. In a series of sessions, I guided Maia through meditations of her pelvis as a sacred space. Reflecting upon her negative body associations, she began to understand that her relationship to her core would change if she perceived her body as sacred.

By choosing to establish a sense of the sacred in her body, Maia was able to clarify her energy patterns. She identified uses of her energy that dishonored her being: patterns of negative self-talk or of ignoring her bodily needs. Maia noticed that she was less respectful to herself when feeling out of balance in her core. Instead of dwelling on her negative patterns, she began to focus on her root and ask herself what she needed. When she did this, she was immediately guided to simple acts of self-care or ways to address an unhealthy situation.

One year later, Maia conceived and gave birth to a daughter. Because she had discovered her own potential for celebrating her female body, she welcomed her daughter joyfully, rather than with fear. After her daughter's birth, Maia realized that the baby would continue to seek nourishment and solace from her body, so in mothering her daughter, she found many opportunities to invite the sacred back to her body.

A mother's body is the physical and energetic anchor for her child. Her relationship to her body will deeply impact her child's sense of self, because that body serves as the beginning place for this child. In addition, communication between a mother and child is primarily nonverbal and also based in the mother's body.

As Maia's connection with her body changed from avoidance and shame to honor and respect, her daughter benefited from this positive shift. Reclaiming the sacred in her body allowed Maia to hold herself and her child in a different way. Doing this work enabled her to make a tremendous gift to herself and her future lineage.

## Your Pelvis as Sacred Space

Creating sacred space, such as an altar, involves intentionally making a particular place to meet with spirit. A designated altar space serves as a reminder of and commitment to making a change or manifestation through the symbolic expressions of your feminine self. It is a direct way to acknowledge your feminine desires and a safe place to mourn your pain as you reshape and begin to honor your femininity.

The dictionary defines *sacred* as "something regarded with or deserving of deep respect." When you think of your pelvis as sacred space, you care for the core of your female body as you would a precious place. When honored, it can bring forth your manifestation of the divine, whether in the form of your own radiance, children, heartfelt work, creative acts, or other representations of your feminine experience.

Visualize your womb space as an altar where you honor your femininity. Bring together your everyday experiences and your spiritual practice, and you will encounter the profound healing and guidance available for your feminine self in the realm of spirit.

## Seek the Sacred

The first step in restoring the sacredness of your body is to ponder your relationship with the sacred. Connecting with the sacred may involve visiting a particular place in nature, gathering with community, or a doing a specific ritual. You may find the sacred in meditation, creation, or song. You may pray, walk, chant, or dance. Seek the sacred in your life and connect it with your femininity. Reflections on seeking the sacred include:

What is sacred to you?
How do you honor the sacred aspects of your life?
How will you celebrate your sacred femininity?

## Return to the Center

Connect with spirit from your own center. Listen to the wisdom that arises from your core. Rather than body image, which comes from an external perspective, cultivate body awareness—an experience of body from the inside out. Meet with others from this internal place. Honor yourself by creating, moving, and unfolding from this sacred center within.

## Nurture the Sacred

To nurture the sacred in your center, first cultivate a sacred space in ways that invoke the sacred for you. Utilize ritual, prayer, art, or whatever speaks to your wild feminine spirit, and then prepare to receive the blessings that arrive. Tending a sacred space in the heart of your female body brings about direct insight, healing, and transformation for your womanhood.

One of my clients used the following exercise for creating sacred pelvic space to clear the energy of abuse from her pelvis. Another client shared it with a group of women friends and found that it sparked an evening of conversation about the joy and shame of being female. I miscarried a child and in the days following the parting of her spirit, I had a vision. I saw many spirits gathered together, the future children of this planet, and felt their desire to inhabit a place of connection, clarity, and sacredness in their mothers. I pray that all women will begin to realize the sacred potential they carry in the root of their bodies. Use the following exercise to visualize this sacred space in your own pelvis.

### Exercise: Creating Sacred Pelvic Space

1. Find a quiet place and read through the exercise before beginning this visualization.

2. Settle into a comfortable position and bring your attention to the center of your pelvic bowl. Notice any sensations, feelings, or qualities regarding your pelvic energy.

3. Clear your pelvic space. Begin by visualizing water pouring over your pelvis or the smudging of sage smoke around you—

cleansing and clearing your pelvic energy. Choose the element you are drawn to and visualize the water or sage moving in a circular pattern and clearing each part of your pelvic bowl.

4. Invite the water to wash into the earth or the smoke to lift into the sky anything that is not serving your body or being. There, in the earth or sky, this energy will be received and recycled; it is no longer needed in your life. Continue until you feel a sense of peace and clarity in your pelvic bowl.

5. Picture your pelvic bowl as an altar space and imagine placing your offerings here. Offerings may include expressions of gratitude for the abundance in your life, requests for support to make changes, images of your creations, or whatever else comes from your feminine spirit.

6. Rest in quiet reflection and pay attention to the words or visions that come to you. Listen for the guidance or comfort that comes in a sacred place.

7. Close your visualization with gratitude for what you have received. Drink a glass of water, take a walk in the fresh air, or put on a vibrant color—something to honor your body. Allow your sacred femininity to inspire your everyday living.

Another way to nurture the sacred in your daily life is to set a bowl on your altar—a symbol of your pelvic bowl—and fill it with words that cherish your femininity. Words, when chosen with intent, are powerful catalysts for transformation. Images can be added as well. Looking at pictures and the visual aspects of the other objects on your altar will engage your unconscious mind and serve as a reminder to celebrate your female form.

To further clear any negative associations or imprints from your body, bless yourself with water or words. I often bless my body in the shower, splashing my skin with loving intent as I bathe. Taking the moments and events that occur daily and making them sacred is a beautiful way to honor yourself and how your feminine is expressed. By using "ordinary" to create ritual, we elevate every day to a blessing for ourselves. Blessing your body is a direct act of healing.

Our beauty shines in the light of spirit. The imprints of pain that we carry in the pelvic bowl can be softened when we bring the blessing energy to our center. Blessings work on the deeper layers to heal our spiritual fractures: these places where we have lost touch with spirit. Blessings are a salve that we can use to restore our inherent wholeness. Write a body blessing, or use the following one, and honor your sacred self.

### Exercise: Body Blessing

*Bless my feet and legs; let them walk with the grounding energy of the earth.*

*Bless my pelvis, that I may hold my values as a woman, make space for my creations, and release what no longer belongs with me.*

*Bless my vagina; may I be clear about what I bring into or release from my body or life.*

*Bless my feminine organs, that I use my creative potential in ways that are beneficial and sustainable for my spirit.*

*Bless my belly; may I be in my place of feminine power.*

*Bless my hands and arms; may they cultivate and receive a joyful bounty.*

*Bless my heart and chest, that I receive and give fully the love I share with others.*

*Bless my breasts, that I nourish myself as lov-*
*ingly as I nourish my creations.*
*Bless my throat and head; may I speak my truth*
*and clarify my visions.*
*Bless the paths behind and ahead of me, that they*
*may transform what I carry into the future.*
*Bless the place I now stand as a woman; may I*
*be fully present in my body and life and cele-*
*brate the blessings of this moment.*

To fully commit to the sacred means clearing space for that which is precious. Cultivating the sacred in your root restores the union between your feminine spirit and female body. Spirit will once again inhabit the ground that is held as sacred; with this potential in your creative center, you receive the blessings made possible in the midst of the divine.

*May you remember your sacred body.*

# FOUR

# Expressing Your Wild Femininity

*The ovaries move the vibrant feminine and masculine energies in
the pelvic bowl so that we can create with balance and beauty in all
that we do. So many of our present-day forms—from personal habits
to the work, political, healthcare, and other structures that shape our
lives—have been constructed with an absence of the feminine and
with a distorted masculine. We all suffer from the lack of more
natural and creative designs. This chapter teaches how to restore
the movement of feminine and masculine energies through
our female bodies so that they will once again flow
through our lives—bringing joy and nurturance
of the soul back to the center where they belong.*

The grass field was wet with rain when we arrived, a rainbow
spread across the purple sky. Now, it is dark. There are stars all
around, and the ground is unexpectedly warm on my bare feet. I am
standing with several others whose faces disappear into the night.
Earlier in the afternoon, as we made a bonfire, the heat pushed us
back from our circle. Several hours have passed since then. In the
darkness, we stand close together, our bodies drawn in toward
the simmering coals. The heat of the fire is softer now, and deeper.
Looking into the pulsing red of this fire, I feel my own energy pulse
in response. It is time for our fire walk.

When I first heard of a fire walk, I thought it must have been
a hoax. Now, after helping build the fire and watching heat rise off

the coals, I know how real it is. Later, I will feel its heat on my bare feet. The fire will burn and threaten to blister the sole of my right foot.

Our guide on this fire walk, a playful woman named Ava, leads us through meditative and physical exercises that prepare us to walk the hot coals. We are matching our energy to the fire's energy. The idea is that fire will not burn that which is like fire. From my work with women, I know that ovaries contain the fire energy of the female body. In my own energy system, I have difficulty warming my right ovary. During our fire walk preparations, my left ovary and left side become fiery and warm. My right ovary and leg remain stiff and wooden.

The first time I walk across the fire bed, my right foot burns. I sit down and remember Ava's warnings. When another firewalker was concerned about being burned, she cautioned him against giving the idea too much energy. She assured him that burns would be treated, telling him to trust his instinct about whether or not to walk across the fire.

I feel the burning on my right foot and think about the energy of fire. As I pay attention to the burn, the sensation of pain intensifies. I am afraid. But I am more afraid of letting my right side become fiery than I am of being burned. I recognize that wooden sensation for what it is: my own attempt to tamp down the inner fire of my right ovary and extinguish the visible fire of my personality.

At the fire's edge, I discover an important distinction. Rather than increase the fire of my right ovary, I need to let go of my tendency to control it. I remember a woman, a participant in one of my classes. We were talking about the ovaries and creative expression when her voice arose in the circle. She said she was tired of living small, of dimming her own radiance. Each woman nodded in agreement.

I decide to let the heat spread from my right foot. This decision feels dangerous. With my permission, the heat shoots upward into my right side. From beneath my initial hesitation, a sense of delight rises to the surface. I take my place at the head of the fire bed and sprint across the coals two more times. Heat rises off my body and out into the black of the night. The heat in my foot dissipates.

In the morning, as soon as I awaken, I search the bottom of my right foot. There, where I felt the burn of the fire, is a red mark. A round, red area in the center of my foot, it is raised slightly like a blister but without pain. The mark is a reminder to tend the creative flame: smoldering fires burn without intention, while tended fires give warmth. My creative fire nourishes me when I move past my fears of being burned and make way for its fiery expression.

## Ovarian Energy and Your Creative Fire

Ovarian energy is a woman's creative fire energy. It is the energetic source of life force energy utilized in making children, as well as making any creation a woman brings into the world. The ovaries are essential for revitalizing a woman's womb. They nourish the female body, and their health determines a woman's radiance.

The ovaries are a woman's best girlfriends. When a woman focuses on the power of her ovaries, she discovers an energy like that created when women talk joyfully together. If a woman directs her attention to one of her ovaries, she inevitably uncovers her craving for something wildly expressive, like leopard-print boots. Because of the power of ovarian energy, many people attempt to harness a woman's creative fire. She may also give away her fire energy, or creative essence, to others. When she exchanges this energy for the promise of security or acceptance, she does not realize its value. A woman's internal flame is intended for her own use.

My own experience of connecting with my ovaries opened my eyes to color. Wearing clothing became a sensory experience; instead of the pale shades I was accustomed to, I began to choose colors and textures each day based on how they inspired my senses. I experimented with full shades of red, then turquoise, bright green, and deep brown. Rather than simply an expression of fashion, clothing became a form of play: a personal and intimate way to relate with my feminine form. Wearing fabrics and colors that enlivened my energy both delighted and honored my body.

To maintain ownership and revel in the warmth of your ovarian energy, know there is choice and power in the way that you use your fire energy. Hold on to your fire, and you will discover your own creative muse.

### Exercise: Reclaim Your Fire Energy

1. Reflection: Begin to reclaim your fire energy by taking charge of your creativity. How are you currently using your creative energy? Does it reflect your true feminine self? Ponder the unique contribution of your heartfelt creations. They serve a purpose in your life and in sustaining the collective feminine nature.

2. Ritual: First, write down three creative sparks, the dream seeds of your wild feminine. Then, write down one action that enlivens each one. When you have finished, light a candle to symbolize your ovarian fire and make the intention to ignite your creative flames.

## Tending the Fire of Your Ovaries

With their limitless potential for creation, the ovaries are a powerful resource in a woman's creative life. A woman with balanced ovarian energy will have an abundance of creative energy to fuel her projects and still be able to nourish herself, even as she creates. Her creations will express her personal visions, and she finds her joy in the process of bringing them to fruition. She will be visibly centered and satisfied, taking her fill of life energy and able to share her radiance with others.

The ovaries hold the receptive fuel and projective power, the cycle of creation, for all a woman's creations. The left and right ovaries work synergistically, alternately recharging or revealing a woman's creative expression. However, they nourish and inspire a woman's creations only when they are in balance.

The energy flow in the body, and the ovaries, moves like a small river. An energetic imbalance occurs in any region of the body where the energy flow, or chi, is higher or lower than is necessary to achieve a balance. If energy is underflowing, it becomes stagnant. If energy is overflowing, it becomes depleted. But if the energy is in a steady, balanced flow, then it is both moved and replenished. *Note*: Even when one or both ovaries have been removed, the energy center associated with the ovary can still be cultivated.

Patterns of ovarian energetic imbalance are almost universal among women, perhaps because we have not learned how to use this powerful energy residing in our female bodies. The ovaries are often overused or blocked in some way, and these energy imbalances, if unaddressed, will impact pelvic health and vitality. They cause pelvic energy stagnation and set the stage for disease or dysfunction in the pelvic space. The vibrancy of your ovarian energy depends on the care you take in tending your creative fire. Reflections on your ovarian fire include:

How are you presently tending your fire?
Are you adding fuel to your fire or heading toward burnout?
Do you sit by the fires you make and receive the warmth
  they offer?

## Sensing Ovarian Energy

With some practice, you will be able to feel your ovarian energy. Although the ovaries are about the size of walnuts, their energy may be perceived as a gentle warmth the size of a small orange in each side of your pelvis. Your ovarian energy can also be sensed externally, as softly radiating warmth from the skin surface to approximately one inch above your skin. Meditating on the ovaries and ovarian energy is the first step in cultivating your creative fire.

Imagine a line from your pubic bone (the bony area just above your vagina) to the crest of your pelvis (the top of your pelvic bowl). Place a hand in the middle of this imaginary line, one on each side of your pelvis. A few inches below each hand lies your right or left ovary. Touch your skin in these regions to sense their energy. Notice if the skin is hot or cold, tight or loose. The sensation over a healthy ovary is moderate warmth covered by soft, pliable skin. Variations may indicate an ovarian energetic imbalance. Working with any imbalances you find, you will also discover how to rekindle your inner fire.

### Exercise: Meditation on the Ovaries

1. Find a comfortable sitting position. Take a moment to sense each of your ovaries. If you feel the warmth of your left ovary in your left pelvis, try to visualize it or sense it with your inner awareness. What do you notice about the energy of your left ovary? Is it hot or cool? Tight or soft? Can you sense the edges of your ovarian energy? Do you see any colors or images? Shift your weight to the left, noticing the whole energetic range on the left side and whether or not you inhabit this full space.

2. Now shift your attention to the right side. Try to both feel and visualize the energy of the right ovary. How does this ovary compare to the left one? Shift your weight to the right; notice the whole energetic range on the right side and whether or not you inhabit this full space.

3. Notice the differences between your ovaries and the energetic range of each side. Left and right ovaries vary in their energetic qualities, but differences in the fullness of their warmth or energy sensations can alert you to an energetic imbalance.

4. Ponder the creative sparks of your ovaries, the vast resources held in these potent organs. Imagine yourself accessing the full radiance and warmth of each ovary.

5. Bring your visualization to a close. Offer gratitude to your ovaries, the source of your creative fire.

### Identify Ovarian Energetic Imbalances and Claim Your Creative Fire

The ovaries replenish and move the energy in the female body, which then impacts how a woman uses creative energy in her daily life. Balanced ovarian energy is essential for a woman to nourish her core, inhabit her full creative range, and fashion a creatively satisfying life.

I have found three primary ovarian energetic imbalances in my work with women: a blocked ovary, an absent ovary, and an overactive ovary. These imbalances can occur in either the right or left ovaries, but because the ovaries work together, an imbalance in one often causes the other to compensate in some way.

> *Blocked ovary:* There is little to no energy flowing in a blocked ovary. This blockage results in excess buildup of energy, creating energetic stagnation and pelvic congestion. Blocked ovaries are often a protective mechanism for shutting down unwanted energy and rejecting aspects of feminine identity. Even as a protective mechanism, however, a blocked ovary prevents a woman from receiving her feminine gifts and using her feminine power. This

pattern creates a sense of internal scarcity because it
blocks potentially nourishing energy as well.

*Absent ovary:* With an absent ovary, the energy is flowing,
   yet the woman is not mindful of its flow. This lack of
   awareness creates an indiscriminate intake or outpouring
   of energy; as a result, a woman feels powerless in some
   way and receives energy indiscriminately. Energy continues to flow through the ovary, but the woman does not
   receive this source of nurturance or power in her own
   life. She may feel victimized, overwhelmed, or confused
   without realizing her own participation in this pattern.

*Overactive ovary:* If the ovary is overactive, the energy is
   flowing in excess and begins to drain a woman's life force.
   The woman with an overactive left ovary is an excessive
   nurturer, taking in too much energy from others and fulfilling their emotional or other needs. As a result, she has
   no space to nourish her own needs. The woman with an
   overactive right ovary is a helper, working tirelessly in the
   outer world. In both cases, the women are often drained
   or depleted and distracted from the core work in their
   own lives.

These different ovarian imbalances have distinct sensations as a
result of the lack or excess energy flow. The energy of a blocked
ovary is dense and small with a hot sensation. The energy of an
absent ovary feels cold or difficult to sense, while the energy of an
overactive ovary is diffuse with unclear boundaries. All these ovarian energetic imbalances are often accompanied by decreased skin
elasticity in the region over the ovary. As the imbalances begin to
impact pelvic health, vitality is diminished and ovarian cysts may
develop.

Unless you have experience with energy or have learned how to sense the energy in your body, the specific energy patterns may be difficult to assess. Assessing your specific pattern is difficult because imbalances can be layered (like an overactive ovary in childhood that is later overwhelmed by the energy and becomes absent) or because there can be different imbalance patterns in different areas of your life (such as overactive in your work life and blocked in intimate relationships). Rather than knowing your specific pattern of ovarian imbalance, it is more essential to know that any ovarian *imbalance* is corrected by ovarian *presence* and awareness of the external patterns that affect creative energy flow. Since the ovaries influence your daily energy use, you may look outside of your body to the external patterns in your life, ways of being or using your creative energy, to discover tendencies toward imbalance. External creative energy patterns both reflect and maintain ovarian imbalances and can provide clues to yours. Working toward a more balanced outer life will also support balance in your core. When you have ovarian balance in your core, you continuously receive warmth from and give expression to your own creative fire.

### Left and Right Ovary: The Feminine–Masculine Connection

To further understand the potential within the ovaries, it is beneficial to explore the distinct left and right ovarian qualities. The left side of the body is related to the feminine or receptive nature, and the left ovary receives energy that inspires and feeds a woman's creative center. The right side of the body is related to the masculine or projective nature, and the right ovary moves a woman's creative energy outward, enabling her to manifest her creative inspirations.

While working in the root of the female body, I frequently witness the unique qualities of the left versus right ovary. These differences can be further examined through the field of neuroscience. The brain is divided into two main lobes, the left and right hemispheres. Each lobe has distinct functions and also relays many of the signals relating to the opposite side of the body. For example, the right side of the brain controls the muscles and movement patterns on the left side of the body. It also regulates images and nonlinear, holistic, and intuitive processes—the feminine realm. The left side of the brain controls the movement patterns on the right side of the body and regulates the written word, logic, and linear processes—the masculine realm. Thus touch, movement, and awareness exercises (such as drawing with the non-dominant hand) can put us in connection with one or the other brain hemisphere, its associated qualities, and ways of using our energy.

Pioneering surgeon and author Dr. Leonard Shlain writes about the differences between the left and right lobes of the brain and the potential for brain structure to influence the culture at large in his book *The Alphabet Versus the Goddess: The Conflict Between Word and Image*. He describes the right side of the brain (left side of the body) as more focused on *being*, and the left side of the brain (right side of the body) as more focused on *doing*. Shlain traveled to the Mediterranean and noticed that the demise of the goddess and the fall of women's status began around the time that people were learning to write, and he hypothesized that perhaps the new skill of writing changed the brain's structure so that the left hemisphere (with its modes of thought and emphasis on doing) was reinforced at the expense of the right hemisphere (and its more feminine values and emphasis on being).

We can translate the same pattern of right body (masculine) and left body (feminine) to the energy of the ovaries: the right ovarian energy relates to *doing* and the left ovarian energy to *being*. I have seen this manifested in many of my clients; when they are focused on the doing or outward expressions of their creative energy, then the right ovary becomes warm and energized (increasing the energy flow in the right side of the pelvic bowl, right breast, and even hand). As they ponder receiving energy, nourishing themselves, and being creative in a nonproductive manner, their left ovary comes to life (bringing more energy to the left breast and left side of the body). However, a woman needs access to both aspects of her energy to be both creative and sustainable, to maintain the health of her body, and to be connected to her creative process in a personal and soulful manner.

In a culture based on production, doing—or right ovarian— activities tend to be more valued than being. Hence, the masculine potential becomes more valuable and predominant than the feminine. Without the feminine, the masculine also becomes distorted. True masculine energy is vibrant and playful, energizing and radiant. Any system based primarily on an imbalanced masculine output is unsustainable, though, because it relies on continual output (doing) without replenishment (being), and it also becomes more punishing and relentless rather than playful.

The imbalance of the masculine and feminine is echoed within the female body through core tension, less engagement, and decreased sensation on one side of the pelvis or the other. Energetically, one of the ovaries may have diminished energy while the other ovary overcompensates. On an emotional and spiritual level, women often have to choose between the outer (masculine) realm and the inner (feminine) realm. All women are challenged to balance the outer and inner callings in their lives—to do work that provides both community or economic value and more internal personal fulfillment. Mothers are more aware of this outer-versus-inner split because they have children who call them back to the womb and the home. Unless they build a new path for themselves, mothers must choose between careers that bring income and recognition or the less tangible rewards of nurturing the family.

## The Lawyer/Mother
A woman having to balance her practice of law with becoming a mother, the lawyer/mother as named by Dick Roy, attorney and

founder of Northwest Earth Institute, epitomizes this struggle between the outer and inner realms. The field of law is logical, clearly defined by principles and based on written words (recorded legal documents that spell out the "letter of the law")—a left-brained profession. Mothering (and most creative work) is intuitive and requires a woman to spontaneously respond to the intimate relationship and primarily visual cues of her infant—an inherently right-brained experience. I have witnessed the struggles of some of these women in my practice, the lawyer/mothers who are challenged by this divide and called to create the necessary bridges to be able to both practice law and mother their children.

One lawyer/mother came to my office with pelvic pain and muscle weakness after the birth of her baby. As I worked on her body, I noticed that all her strength and vitality was on the right side, the masculine. I brought her attention to the imbalance between her right and left, the split in her pelvis. She noted that her body echoed the split in her life. It was difficult for her to be a mother (or to embody the feminine) because she never felt that her own mother was valued.

As a young woman, she had deliberately aligned herself with her father. Cutting her hair short and pursuing a degree in law (like her father had) were direct attempts for validation. She was aware of her desire for validation but did not know that this split was carried within her own body. Likewise, her present-day life was still bound by this separation. With tears in her eyes, she told me of her plans to go back to work and "do less mothering" because after nine months of staying home with her baby, she felt "devalued." Her body was still only geared for external validation, yet she yearned for something deeper.

## New Feminine-Masculine Forms

Mothers are acutely aware of the masculine/feminine divide, but until we make new feminine-masculine forms the whole community is living with less. The more we value external output (doing) that has no relation to our creative needs and potential, we not only establish an unsustainable practice, but we also leave a void in the inner realm (our place of being). Women are the energy keepers. They take energy in (seeds, food, raw material) and they put it out into form (children, meals, medicine) to sustain the tribe. In this way, a woman moves in a continuous cycle, from feminine nourishment to masculine form. She sows seeds and grows her crop. All women carry this earth cycle in their wombs, the place from which life emerges.

As cultures move away from a community model, the awareness for this earth-and-womb cycle decreases. Women's inner power and the value in their bodies are diminished. Women even perceive the menstrual cycle as a burden, rather than as the tidal flow that sustains life. From an early age, girls know their choices: align with the more feminine roles and surrender external value, or step into a career that promises to maintain value but requires relinquishing the feminine. When women come to my office for care, I see these compromises manifest as physical and energetic imbalances within the pelvic bowl. All women (and men) are living with the masculine/feminine split. Wherever a woman has given up her creative ground, I find divisions in the core of her body.

The only way to heal the masculine/feminine split that presently continues to define our lives is to return to the female body. To realign with earth-centered values as a community, women must listen to the earth cycle within themselves. When a woman makes creative choices based on the wisdom of her womb, these choices are more likely to be sustainable, organic, and joy-filled. With guidance from the womb, some lawyer/mothers might turn toward the home and restore an internal sense of value for themselves. Others would bring their feminine vitality into the profession of law and create a human-centered practice, such as a more creative team approach and less demanding schedules; each woman would make the best life for herself and her creations.

There are many paths to make new feminine-masculine forms, and as gender roles continue to fall away, we need to call upon our internal and bodily resources to continue the evolution. By addressing the imbalances within ourselves, we can change unsustainable patterns in our cores that relate to the feminine and masculine. Both left and right ovaries and their feminine and masculine energy potential bring abundance to our creative lives as women. When we understand the intrinsic value of both our feminine and masculine energies, we may learn where to stoke or rekindle these internal flames so that our lives will truly sustain us.

## Left Ovary: Muse and Receptive Nature

The left ovary is the energetic place of receiving whatever a woman desires for her feminine self. It is a woman's inner muse, bringing in her unique sense of beauty, sensuality, and other personal interpretations of the feminine.

The left ovary plugs directly into the true feminine, regenerating creativity and connecting a woman to the abundance of spirit and her feminine lineage. This is also the place a woman must be present to consciously choose what energy and experiences she receives into her body and life. In my work with women who seek to connect with this ovary, issues frequently arise involving feminine identity, pelvic boundaries, and ownership of one's femininity and female body.

When the left ovary is blocked, a woman may identify with an externally defined femininity rather than one derived from her own imagination. For example, a woman dresses or acts in the manner that she perceives to be appropriate, taking cues from outside sources rather than what appeals to her own sense of color and expression. Or a woman may reject the appearances or roles that she perceives as feminine. I often hear women bemoan the princess parties that their young daughters are excited about. Yet the soft fabrics, sparkly trim, and dreamy qualities of a princess are quite feminine. In either case, whether a woman conforms to or rejects a prescribed femininity, she is reacting to her feminine identity rather than making it her own authentic creation. As women access the left ovary, they tap into their own feminine energy and become newly inspired. The muse in the left ovary simply enjoys her own idea of beauty.

The left ovary contains a playful essence that is frequently undervalued in a culture fixated on production. Listening to the wisdom of this ovary, a woman hears a voice saying, *Let's take a bath, daydream, and be timeless, or get dressed up for no particular reason other than the joy of it.* Taking time for seemingly frivolous indulgences is essential to replenishing the energy of the left ovary that sustains a woman's spirit and, ultimately, fuels her external work.

When fully present in the left ovary, you are able to both receive and claim your feminine nature. You create your own definition of what it means to be a woman, and you choose the elements of your feminine lineage that you desire. You cultivate your creative potential, intuition, and other feminine gifts for use in your own life. You embody the beauty of your full and vibrant femininity. Reflections regarding the left ovary include:

How do you currently experience the feminine?
With your receptive capacities, are you receiving anything that does not serve you?
How do you nourish your creative center?
What is the essence of your left-ovary energy, and how do you access it in your life?

## Left-Ovary Imbalances
In order to nourish herself while using her creative energy and to ensure that her creations reflect her personal vision, a woman must

have balanced energy flow in her left ovary. Since women rarely access the feminine, their creative lives are often shaped by external structures such as gender expectations, income needs, workplaces, and professions that often poorly serve women and their creations—which further disparages the feminine. As the primary connection to the feminine realm, the left ovary suffers from many imbalances relating to the denigration and subsequent disappearance of the feminine. To restore balance in our lives, we need the feminine. However, it is essential to have feminine energy running through our bodies before it can return to our lives.

Receiving the feminine into the body provides inspiration for changing the structures that place limitations on gender roles, personal value, creative vitality, and the balance between outer work and inner home. The experiences of women in the stories that follow bear witness to the ways ovarian imbalances affect our daily energy intake. These stories illustrate how women access or inadvertently block the feminine in their bodies and how this influences the shape of their lives. They provide us a greater understanding of the true potential for transformation that becomes available when we receive the warmth of the left ovary, this inner fire of our wild feminine.

## Blocked Left Ovary: Rejecting Feminine Receptive Power

One of the most common ovarian energetic imbalances is a blocked left ovary, in which a woman rejects her feminine receptive power. Power is typically thought of as an external force, but the feminine power to receive and transform energy is an often overlooked yet profound type of power.

The female body receives energy through the left ovary, but it is also the place a woman tightens to block energy she does not want to receive, including the energy of people or experiences that are toxic to her feminine self. However, attempting to block energy is as futile as stopping a flow of water. It requires a continuous effort to hold the blockage in place, and some of the energy still flows around it. This defense mechanism ultimately leaves a woman vulnerable to receiving others' negative energy because her attention is focused on what she is trying to block.

Likewise, when a woman's feminine spirit conflicts with familial or cultural aspects of feminine identity, she may tighten her body and again block the left, or receptive, ovary as a protective response. However, decreased access to the left ovary results in external patterns of living that do not reflect a woman's feminine nature or creative gifts. If a woman blocks the receptive ovary to reject limiting ancestral or cultural aspects of feminine identity, she also blocks her own receptive powers. Decreased access to the left ovary restricts her creative inflow and ability to replenish her energy.

A woman may have blocked her left ovary as a protective response or as a result of wounding related to her femininity, power, creativity, or sensual expression. If a woman believes she cannot be both feminine and powerful, she may have felt the need to choose between her left and right ovarian powers. The flow of feminine energy is what gives a woman her vibrancy, but if her experiences have shown her that it is unsafe to be visible or sensual, she may block her bodily access to feminine energy. However, true protection arises from a woman's solid presence in the left ovary. Reflections regarding a blocked left ovary include:

How have you restricted your capacity for receiving feminine inspiration or energy?
What is needed to replenish your creative center and wild feminine self?

*Women's Stories: Receiving Sustenance from the Feminine*

Mary came to my office to restore balance in her pelvic bowl. She had an overall sense of bodily fatigue and depletion that was noticeably worse during menstruation, and she wondered if bodywork might alleviate her symptoms. While reviewing her intake forms, I noticed that her torso had a subtle twist pattern, so that her upper body was turned away from her left side, and she had an energetic blockage in the left side of her pelvis. I mentioned the body pattern to Mary, and she told me that her left ovary had been removed ten years previously because of a cyst.

The energy blockage in Mary's left pelvis may have contributed to the formation of an ovarian cyst. Physical symptoms often arise in the places where blocked energy creates stagnation. Even though an ovary (or uterus) is removed, the organ energy is still present and can be accessed in the pelvis. Mary and I talked about the importance of the receptive energy in her left side and its connection to her overall health. As I began the bodywork portion of our session, I encouraged her to focus on her left pelvis and the region of her left ovary.

Mary had difficulty paying attention to the left side of her body. As we worked together, she noticed her inclination to focus on the right side instead. Women with a greater focus on the right side of the body tend to accomplish task upon task, because the right ovary is on the masculine side of the body and relates to the outer world. This imbalance makes a woman extremely productive, but it depletes her energy system and leaves little time for any left ovarian activities—the replenishment activities that do not appear to serve a tangible purpose.

As I described the difference between the right and left ovaries, and patterns of imbalance, Mary could relate to the description of a dominant right ovary and a blocked left ovary. She was an activist and felt compelled to work long hours; the importance and intensity of her work never allowed time for activities that felt unproductive. Though she loved books, with

a pile of unending tasks awaiting her attention, it seemed frivolous to sit down and read.

I asked Mary to imagine herself doing her activist work
while observing her ovarian energy. In doing so, she noticed
that her right ovary seemed exhausted while the region around
her left ovary felt constricted. Mary realized that no matter
how much energy she gave, there was still work to do. Her
body was overwhelmed by the endless demands of her work,
and she recognized the irony of trying to set up sustainable
systems in the outer world while continuously depleting her
own body.

I invited Mary to imagine herself in a relaxed state,
perhaps settling into her favorite chair with a good book.
When she did this, Mary noticed that her left ovary became
soft and warm. The difference was dramatic. Meanwhile, her
right ovary felt as if it was in a deep and restful sleep. Allowing
herself the satisfaction of a seemingly unproductive activity
resulted in a profound rebalancing of Mary's core energy.

As Mary felt the restored energetic balance in her body, she
realized that she had been operating from a place of imbalance
for years. Her own mother was a stay-at-home mom, whose
work in the home kept her continuously busy. Mary never felt
that her mother enjoyed mothering, and she had intentionally
established a career she was passionate about in order to make a
different life for herself. Ironically, in her pattern of continual
doing, she was using her creative energy in the same way as her
own mother. Mary had changed the outer structure of her life
by working outside of the home, but she continued the same
internal energy pattern because she was always busy and did
not allow herself to enjoy the fruits of her labor.

Mary chose a meaningful career, seeking the satisfaction
that was missing in her mother's life. Yet even in the home,
Mary's mother could have focused on the left, receptive side of

her body to savor the delight contained within every day. This connection would have changed her mothering and Mary's experience as her daughter. Somewhere in their maternal lineage, women blocked the left ovary and their ability to receive delight from simple, daily pleasures. Mary may never know what created this energetic imbalance, but she can still address it in order to reform her own experience as a woman. Whether a woman is tending children or a demanding career, it is essential to stay aware of the left ovary so that she is sure to receive, even as she gives, energy. With a connection to the feminine in her body, she will be more likely to rest as needed, say no to extra demands, or recharge herself in the midst of her daily life.

In working with the energy of the ovaries, I have observed that the left ovary contains the capacity for a woman to take in the sustenance of the moment. The right ovary creates and builds, but the left ovary is the source of this inspiration. Together they enable a woman to both make and partake from her creative abundance. Changing an ovarian imbalance often requires a woman to transform the lineage patterns that govern how she accesses the creative energy in her root.

In blocking the energy of her left ovary, Mary was also blocking her potential to receive her feminine nourishment. Unable to replenish herself and continually putting energy outward, Mary was depleted, and a continual depletion without refill results in pelvic energetic imbalance, decreased energy, and eventual illness. Mary's fatigue was preventing her from continuing a high level of activity. In various ways, her body was trying to communicate the necessity of changing her pattern of constant energy use.

To fashion her energy patterns in a more sustainable manner, Mary might look to a role model like Starhawk, a globally known social justice activist who incorporates the feminine realms of ritual and earth-based spirituality directly into her activism. Starhawk credits the creative power of connection to spirit as critical in her ability to have sustained a long-term role as an activist where many others have suffered burnout. Bringing the feminine into any action expands the potential for creation because it draws upon a greater energy from the realm of spirit.

By taking time for the invitations of the left ovary, Mary would find the sustenance readily available in each day. By allowing the energetic flow in this left ovary, she would also transform the inherited pattern of her lineage. Receiving the gifts of the feminine would not only bring nourishment for Mary, but also offer the material for her to reinvent her womanhood, a fresh source of inspiration.

## Absent Left Ovary: Letting Others Steal Your Fire

In the case of an absent left ovary, a woman receives her femininity but then lets others take possession of this fire energy for their own needs. This ovarian energetic pattern is often present in women with relationship power imbalances. A woman with an absent left ovary may passively receive uninvited sexual attention, continue to work in a job where she is being taken advantage of, or repeatedly allow external circumstances to define her present life.

Women from female lineages that are highly intuitive but who unconsciously reject this ability may use the pattern of an absent ovary as a protective response. Ironically, though their intent is to reject their inherent intuitiveness, they leave themselves wide open to it because the left ovary continues energetically receiving emotional energy or other subtle energies without their conscious presence. Reflections regarding an absent left ovary include:

What creative abilities or parts of your feminine range have you let go of?

How might you restore these gifts for yourself?

*Women's Stories: Reclaiming the Beauty of Her Feminine*

Melissa sought pelvic work to enhance her feminine connection. Her medical history contained several left-sided body ailments including multiple left ankle sprains, a left wrist fracture, and two left ovarian cysts. An examination of Melissa's pelvic floor revealed significant pelvic weakness on the left side and only a trace of energetic presence in the region of her left ovary.

I directed Melissa's attention to her left ovary, and it was difficult for her to sense its energy. When I asked her to notice what she felt internally, she said it seemed as if she was avoiding the left side of her body. She perceived her right ovary as a small light but noticed that her left ovary seemed cold and isolated.

Using focused breathing and visualization of the left ovary, Melissa became more aware of her left side, and I felt the warmth in her left pelvis and ovary increase significantly. Melissa said that she saw a light in her left ovary; it was slowly growing and filling up the empty space in her pelvis, and then she noticed that her left pelvis felt warmer and more alive but that it still did not feel like a part of her body.

I assured Melissa that this was her rightful place, but I agreed that she was not occupying her full pelvic bowl with her body awareness. Then I explained the role of the left ovary in choosing what energy she received from others and in protecting her energetic space. She told me that she had difficulty protecting herself and frequently experienced unwanted male attention from both work clientele and personal friends. Melissa tried to ignore this attention but was often told that she was "being cold" when she did not respond.

As we talked, Melissa remembered that other female family members, including her mother, sister, and aunt, had shared similar experiences of unwanted male attention. They seemed equally helpless to prevent these situations. Melissa noted that women in her family were also singled out and praised for their external beauty, and while she did not like her appearance to be the focus of attention, Melissa had never felt herself valued by her family for any other qualities.

Every culture identifies and honors that which is deemed beautiful. But this notion of beauty becomes distorted when it is considered something to own, rather than the unique essence of each individual. In Western cultures, men are often denied their own expression of beauty because it is perceived as unmasculine. Yet it is an inherent desire of the feminine nature to share one's beauty with others.

One day, after riding on an old-fashioned merry-go-round, my three-year-old son exclaimed, "Wasn't I beautiful, Mama?" The beauty of his own free spirit exhilarated him. As boys become men, they find their own experience of beauty significantly limited. In response to these wounds to their feminine spirit, men may look to a woman's radiance and attempt to own or dominate her. Male attention that imparts value and ownership of beauty exacts a high price: a woman must give up her feminine ground in exchange for external validation, betraying her wild feminine in the process.

In Melissa's case, avoiding her left pelvis diminished her pelvic energetic boundaries. A woman who is not present in her left ovary may find herself regularly feeling invaded as she receives energy without realizing it. Her body language unconsciously conveys that she is unguarded, and this energetic void on her left signals to others that she is not protecting herself and that, if approached, she will give up her own space.

Since girls often mimic the energetic patterns of their mothers, it is not surprising that Melissa and other women in her family have had common experiences of feeling victimized.

The women of her lineage were leaving themselves energetically unguarded. This is not their fault and in no way blames them for receiving any direct or subtle abuse. However, in self-defense classes, women are taught that a more upright and solid posture offers some protection because it conveys non-verbally to would-be attackers that a woman will stand her ground. In the same manner, when a woman increases the strength of her energetic core, she claims her space and will effectively decrease the amount of unwanted attention she receives.

In addition to the protection provided by a solid presence in the left ovary, being present in this place is essential for a woman to have a healthy relationship with beauty. The terrain of the left ovary is her personal connection to the energy of the feminine that will fulfill and delight her. She brings this energy into her body and is more deeply inspired by the color and texture that surrounds her, with a growing desire to express and engage with beauty as an energy and aesthetic form.

Melissa began to transform her pelvic pattern by bringing her presence to the left ovary on a daily basis, but she realized how uncomfortable she felt inhabiting this part of herself—even when no longer serving us, old patterns are familiar. So she began a daily practice of focusing on her left side each morning in the shower and breathing toward her left ovary to change her habitual pattern of giving up her feminine range. She noticed that this practice increased her ability to feel the shower water flowing over her skin on the left side of her body.

Melissa also visualized the warmth and light of her left ovary when challenged by unwanted attention or other experiences causing her to retreat from her left pelvis. She found that this simple shift in energetic awareness increased her presence in her body and alerted her more quickly to energy that she might be receiving unintentionally. In this way, Melissa was reclaiming her full pelvic space and sending a clear message about her rightful ownership of her radiance. As she allowed herself to receive this feminine energy, she noticed a sense of wonder returning to her days. Melissa recognized that she had been missing the very substance that gives depth and energy to life: the beauty of her own feminine.

## Overactive Left Ovary: Nurturing Beyond the Call of Duty

The left ovary receives energy in the female body, facilitating a woman's ability to nurture others. By drawing in and holding the energy of another, a woman may receive her partner in lovemaking, sustain her child in utero and beyond, or gestate a creative venture. A woman's nurturing capacity is a valuable asset, but it is frequently overused. With an overactive left ovary, a woman may receive too much energy from others, so that she lacks fuel for her own nourishment and project ventures.

Women who take in more energy than they have reserves for may do so because they feel obligated to cater to others or they tend to dismiss their own needs. This energetic imbalance may also be maintained by the belief that a woman's value is connected to the care she provides for others. Her ability to nourish her creations is only sustainable if she nourishes herself as well. Reflections regarding an overactive left ovary include:

What creations are you presently nurturing?
How are you nurturing yourself?

*Women's Stories: Transforming a Pattern of Emotional Caretaking*

Ina sought to resolve symptoms of pelvic heaviness and came in for a pelvic evaluation. Her exam revealed significant tension in the left side of her pelvic muscles. Her left ovarian energy was hot and dry, indicating a pattern of overuse. Ina's internal sense of her left ovary was that it felt very full.

I asked Ina to focus on her left ovary, and immediately several members of Ina's family came to her mind. As the eldest daughter of five children, whose mother struggled with severe mental illness, Ina had become the caretaker for her family at an early age, but as an adult, she had recognized that this role drained her energy. In the past few years, she worked to change the pattern of continuing to serve as the emotional center for her siblings. By observing her left ovary, Ina realized that she was still unintentionally expending her female energy on taking care of her family and unclear about her own needs or boundaries.

We form many early energy patterns in response to our family experiences. A family who loses a parent, either to death or disease, will experience profound and overwhelming emotions. When the parent has been the family nurturer, the children look to another person, often a female, to continue providing the nurturance they require. Ina was able to fulfill this role but did so only to meet the needs of her siblings. This pattern of taking responsibility for others before she was even grown herself was taking its toll on her health. It was time for her to rest by halting her caretaking and using her creative energy for her own life. Just as her body provided guidance about the energy patterns that were draining to her, it also offered direction about how to change these patterns.

When a woman changes the energetic patterns in her core, it is deeply transformative for her life. By changing the way that she uses her creative energy to care for herself and others, she effectively rewrites the unspoken rules that govern the manifestation of her creative impulses. She finds a new potential, greater access to her own feminine essence, and the freedom to direct her joy, her power.

First, Ina needed to release her core sense of responsibility about mothering her siblings. Paying attention to the center of her pelvic bowl, her womb, she recognized her reluctance to give up this duty. She knew her siblings were adults, but with the creative energy of her body, she was still operating as their mother. When she imagined herself as a girl, taking on the weight of mothering before she was grown, Ina felt respect and compassion for the strength of her young self. Ina took a breath and gave herself permission to let go. She exhaled, each time releasing the energy from her core.

Ina's center became hot, the mark of a significant release, and her left leg shook as she surrendered the burden she had carried. After several minutes, her uterine release was complete. Ina remarked on the spaciousness of her left side and the quiet warmth in her ovary. By clearing the emotional energy of responsibility toward her siblings, Ina felt the newly available capacity in her energy system. The tension in her left pelvic muscles was gone.

By changing her core pattern of caretaking, Ina freed herself from unconsciously taking in the energy of others. Now, when faced with family or friends in emotional distress, she can bring awareness to her pelvic bowl. Having released her early imprint of caretaking responsibility, she can make a clear choice about whether or not to use her energetic capacity. Ina will be able to assess her own needs for self-care by bringing her attention to the intuitive left ovary—enabling her to support those around her but also make a conscious choice to support herself as well.

### Exercise: Meditating on the Left Ovary

After learning about patterns of imbalance in the left ovary, meditate on your own left ovary and receptive nature.

1. Bring awareness to the left side of your pelvic bowl, to the left ovary. Pay attention to the sensations you experience. Notice whether the ovary is tight and hot, cold and difficult to sense, diffuse with unclear boundaries, or soft and warm in your pelvic bowl.

2. If you find an imbalance, ask this ovary how to restore your presence here and to receive or replenish your creative energy. Pay attention to images or sensations that arise. How do you connect with the left ovary? Do you engage in any activities that seem to increase the sensation of energy flow or light on the left side of your pelvis? Breathe toward this ovary and invite it to expand its warmth into the full energetic range of the left side. Notice the increase in ovarian warmth and how this feels to your body and your creative flow.

3. Bring your visualization to a close and offer thanks to your left ovary, the inspiration for your creative fire.

## Right Ovary: Cowgirl and Projective Nature

The right ovary is the source of a woman's projective nature, responsible for the direction and manner in which she puts her creations out into the world. It gives her the energy to fix what is broken, protect what is valuable, and forge paths for others to follow. A woman's own inner cowgirl, the right ovary is the explorer of new frontiers who says, *Let's ride.*

The energy of the right ovary is visible in a woman's external roles. This is the place a woman must be present in order to actively choose how she spends time manifesting her purpose in life. In my work with women to connect with this ovary, I have found that it relates to issues involving career, female roles, and ownership of one's creative capacity.

When a woman listens to the wisdom of this ovary, she hears a voice saying, *Go out and make your voice heard. Gather your tools and begin your work. Be bold and brave because your offering is essential.* This voice seems to correspond with the values of a work-oriented culture, yet it speaks not just about paid employment, but about the work of a woman's feminine spirit. The right ovary has the energy to bring a woman's spiritual creations into physical being.

When you fully access the right ovary, your presence is noticeable in the external world: you are able to hold your feminine ground and direct your creative potential. You may call on this ovary to build your creative dreams. Bringing your own expression of femininity into your creations, you are part of the next evolution of feminism, in which women integrate the feminine into all aspects of their personal and work lives. Reflections regarding your right ovary include:

What are you creating in your life as a woman?
How are you directing your creative potential?
How do your creations reflect your unique feminine expression?
What is the essence of your right ovarian energy and how is
   it expressed in your life?

## Right Ovarian Imbalances

To use her creative abilities and shape her creations, a woman must have balanced energy flow in her right ovary. Since the feminine is out of balance in the female body and the predominant culture, women are not receiving the nurturance they need to fuel their outer work. They run their right ovarian energy in a state of perpetual exhaustion, or they shut down the visible nature of this ovary if holding power seems unsafe. The masculine models that influence work, gender roles, and the support available for family life are often set up without regard for the feminine, and women's bodies continue to reflect this masculine/feminine divide.

By examining the imbalances in the right ovary, a woman's connection to the masculine realm, we witness the way these imbalances affect energy output on a daily basis. The stories that follow illustrate how women misuse or inadvertently block the masculine flow in their bodies and lives. Learning how others have worked to change these imbalances inspires us to reclaim and give form to the infinite expression contained within the right ovary, this outer fire of our wild feminine.

## Blocked Right Ovary: Rejecting Projective Masculine Power

When a woman does not make space for her creative projects in the world, either because she undervalues her abilities or simply does not recognize her contributions, she may have an energetically blocked right ovary.

A woman may block her right ovary because she lacks self-worth, feels that having the power to direct her creative energy is unsafe, or because the opportunities she sees before her do not match the desires of her spirit. This woman does not bring her personal vision to the projects she is involved in. Or she may settle for what she gets and decide not to have children, a creative life, a vibrant marriage, or a satisfying career because she lacks faith in her ability to create what she truly wants. A woman may believe she has no right to claim her creative expression. This unclaimed energy ultimately limits a woman's wild feminine range. Reflections regarding a blocked right ovary:

Have you compromised any of your creative visions?
What support do you need to restore your full ability to
   direct your creative energy?

### Women's Stories: Breaking Down the Barriers

Barbara came for pelvic work to restore the balance in her pelvic bowl. An evaluation of her pelvic floor musculature showed increased tension on her right side and a blockage in the energy of her right ovary. Bringing her awareness to the right side of her pelvis, Barbara felt as if a wall blocked the energy flow of her right ovary.

She attempted to visualize her right ovary and sense its warmth, but at first could not see or feel anything except tension. I redirected her attention to the left side, and she was able to feel the warmth of her left ovary. By moving her attention from the left and then back to the right, Barbara practiced sensing the energy of both her ovaries.

Barbara had never focused on her pelvis in this way, and she remarked that her right side felt "stuck." As she said this, she remembered the words she had used recently to describe herself to her husband and close friends. She had been telling them that she felt "stuck" in her life, but did not know what to do about it.

I asked her to bring awareness to the region of her right ovary and look for the place where her energy was stuck. As Barbara did this, a thought came to her. Though she wanted to direct the creative energy in her life, she often felt inhibited. From childhood, she let external circumstances define her and had carried this pattern into her present day life. In the early years of her marriage, she and her husband traveled across the country and experienced the freedom and passion of these times. Now, with the constraints of a home and predictable schedule, her marriage and daily life had fallen into a tedious routine.

I asked her to envision a place where she was free to express her creative energy. Her current job came to mind, where she had developed a position that fit her skills and with colleagues who engaged and challenged her. Her right ovarian energy began to flow, and she felt this warmth in her pelvis. But as she pondered her attempts at domestic tasks, like cooking, and some of the challenges in her marriage, she felt the right ovarian energy diminish. Barbara recognized her tendency to use her outer fire in a singular manner. The discrepancy between what she wanted and what she believed she could have restricted her pelvic energy and her ability to create. As she recognized this limiting pattern, she realized that in many areas of her life, her expectations were for scarcity rather than possibility. When she consciously acknowledged these self-imposed limitations, Barbara's core energy began to change.

She focused on the right ovary, challenging the wall in her body, the barrier of beliefs that blocked her true potential. Barbara directed breath toward her right ovary, asking her body to make space for what she desired in the energetic realm. She created a vision of herself having more energy in the home and greater passion in her marriage. Sensing the wall around her right ovary, she invited her feminine spirit to expand beyond this wall that limited her expression with old beliefs and outdated models of living. As she pushed through the barrier restraining her creative energy, Barbara's body and external life received the full radiance of her outer fire.

## Absent Right Ovary: Giving Away Your Fire

The energetic imbalance of an absent right ovary occurs when a woman uses her creative energy but fails to maintain ownership of her creative direction. Women who are challenged by being seen and recognized as successful, stepping into their authentic identity, or standing up for themselves and the value of what they create often experience this imbalance. A woman with this pattern may sabotage herself or downplay her success to avoid receiving direct attention. She may also relinquish her creative essence in exchange for personal validation and a sense of security or steal the fire of others because she is not building one of her own. A woman will not be able to shine until she sits in the light of her own fire. Reflections regarding an absent right ovary include:

What creative endeavors have you let go of or left unfinished?
What compelled you to abandon your creative form?
Are there any creative aspirations you desire to reclaim?

*Women's Stories: The Woman Who Wanted to Write*

Cora came to me to address postpartum healing from two childbirths. She was exhausted and challenged by her daily demands of mothering. An evaluation of her pelvic floor showed a high level of tension in her muscles and a decreased energetic presence in her right ovary. She had a history of right ovarian cysts.

Guiding Cora to her right ovary, I asked her to be alert for any sensations she noticed. She said that her body felt heavy on the right side; focusing there, she saw an image of herself writing. She explained that her college major was creative writing. She remembered how much she enjoyed writing poetry as a young woman, but her formal education had included a high level of critique; as a result, she began to fear failure and lost the joy in simply creating. During this time, Cora began to have ovarian cysts.

Cora's right ovarian energy was actively involved in the creative process of writing. However, because the external support and validation Cora desired was unavailable, she had stopped writing and curtailed an essential part of her self-expression. The appearance of ovarian cysts may have been her body's attempt to communicate the ovarian energetic imbalance that began as she restricted the flow of creative energy. Cora said that now she devoted herself to motherhood.

Her days were spent taking care of her children, with more of
a sense of duty than joy.

Whenever a woman's feminine identity arises from obligation or need rather than her own desire, it negatively impacts
her creations and creative energy. Likewise, when a woman
clings to the role of mother as her sole identity, she often unintentionally and unconsciously holds her children back from
their own potential. When she mothers in this way, dutifully
but forgoing her own creative impulses, a woman's sense of
self requires the continued dependence of her children. The
true desires of her creative essence go unrecognized.

Cora was using her ovarian energy to nourish her
children but denying the expression of her feminine spirit in
the artistic medium it yearned for. In a situation like hers,
resentment arises at some level and children become aware of
it. This is confusing to them: on one hand, they observe their
mother holding fast to her role as nurturer; but on the other
hand, they sense that her spirit is not fully aligned with this
role. Because her creative energy was not flowing in a sustainable manner, Cora would continue to be depleted by taking
care of her children without regard for herself. And it would
also ultimately prevent her from giving her children an
important gift: without observing their mother honoring herself, they would be less likely to honor her, other women,
or themselves.

Any activity that replenished Cora as a woman would
enhance her mothering in several ways. Because writing is a
passion for her, it would bring fullness to her life and encourage the expansion of her spirit. It would also offer a separate
identity for her, which would allow for her children's independent growth. As Cora made space for her dreams, she
would encourage her children to reach their own potential.
They would observe their mother fulfilling her desires rather

than living with unaddressed needs. Making time for her creative writing would also revitalize the energy of Cora's left and right ovaries by providing a form of internal nurturance and external expression.

## Overactive Right Ovary: A Pattern of Overextension

The energetic imbalance of an overactive right ovary occurs when a woman takes on more projects than she can energetically sustain. Accessing her ovarian energy without replenishing or nourishing herself, she becomes overextended and depletes her energy system. I often find with this pattern that the right pelvis is held slightly forward, as if a woman is about to take a step. Her body reflects the way that she carries herself in the world—with constant activity and little time to sit back onto her pelvic bowl and rest.

An overactive right ovary may develop when a woman believes she must take care of others' physical needs or the external demands of her life in order to be loved or considered worthwhile. Young girls learn this pattern from cultural cues encouraging them to be cooperative and helpful. As a result, they seek validation through what they do for others rather than from what they can create for themselves. A woman's creative work is an essential component of her feminine radiance and manifestation of joy. Reflections regarding an overactive right ovary include:

Are you making time for your own creative endeavors?
How do you value your own sustenance and capacity for creation?

*Women's Stories: Restoring a Sense of Self-Value*

Nancy came for pelvic work to increase her overall energy, as she felt creatively adrift and disconnected from her center. Though she was involved in many aspects of her community, nothing inspired her for more than a brief time. An evaluation of her pelvis revealed diminished energy in her pelvic bowl, difficulty engaging her pelvic floor, and an overactive right ovary.

As I guided Nancy's attention to her ovaries, she reported distinct differences in their sensations. She noticed warmth in her left pelvis, from the left ovary, but found that her right ovary was hard to locate—it did not have clearly defined boundaries like the left. She was describing a typical sensation for an overactive energetic pattern in which the ovarian energy is diffuse and undefined.

By paying attention to her right ovary, Nancy said that she could visualize its energy, like streams of light, going to the various projects she had taken on. Her internal pelvic floor had several areas of tension and tenderness on the right side. This increased noticeably as she described feeling obligated to give her energy away.

I instructed Nancy in a breathing and visualization exercise in which she guided her ovarian energy back to her own body and into her right pelvis. We discussed the powerful energy that her ovaries contained for her. During this exercise, Nancy found herself initially resisting, but then she realized it was because she did not feel worthy to receive the entire focus of her energy.

Nancy was voicing a common lack of self-value among women, one that manifests itself in several ways. For Nancy, becoming involved in multiple activities gave her a sense of meaning and self-worth. She felt obligated to give her creative energy away because she based her personal value on what she did for others, rather than on who she was. She needed to be productive in order to feel purposeful, which did not allow her to feel valuable while resting. Other women respond to a lack of self-value by blocking the left ovary or their ability to take in self-nurturance. Like Nancy, they feel unworthy to receive sustenance for themselves as individuals.

Nancy was motivated to change this pattern of overactivity when she recognized the energetic effects of compromising herself. Taking stock of her energy system, she made a commitment to address her needs for rest and rejuvenation. By bringing her ovarian energy back toward her own being, she not only nourished herself, she also reaffirmed her value. When women honor themselves, they teach others to honor them as well.

### Exercise: Meditating on the Right Ovary

After learning about patterns of imbalance in the right ovary, meditate on your own right ovary and projective nature.

1. Bring awareness to the right side of your pelvic bowl, to the right ovary. Pay attention to the sensations you experience. Notice whether the ovary is tight and hot, cold and difficult to sense, diffuse with unclear boundaries, or soft and warm.

2. If you find an imbalance, ask this ovary how better to express or give form to your creative energy. Pay attention to images or sensations that arise. How do you connect with the right ovary? Do you engage in activities that seem to increase the sensation of energy flow or light on the right side of your pelvis? Breathe toward this ovary and invite it to expand its warmth into the full energetic range of the right side. Feel the increased warmth in the ovary, and the response in your body and your creative flow.

3. Bring your visualization to a close and offer thanks to your right ovary, the visible expression of your creative fire.

## Sadness: Reveal Your Radiance

When a woman lives in the light of her creative fire, her radiance knows no bounds. People notice her, yet her radiance does not depend on their attention. Warmed by her own fire, she is free to share this warmth with others. However, women are often taught to dampen their fire, resulting in the lingering sadness that is the sign of an unrealized potential. Every woman is a fertile and creative being. If her creative impulses remain undeveloped, she will experience a deep sense of loss until she makes and basks in the glow of her own creative fire.

### The Root Voice of Sadness: Unresolved Loss

Each time you encounter sadness in your pelvic space or in regard to your femininity, you have discovered a place of unresolved loss. The root voice of sadness expresses the depth of this loss by saying: *I will never be able to receive or create what I want or I cannot be who I am.*

Wherever a woman is devalued or not received for being her true self, she may foster a mode of protection rather than connection. Rather than risk sharing her expression, a woman shuts down her creative potential. In trying to shield herself from further pain, she inadvertently cuts herself off from her creative essence and denies herself the experience of fulfilling her creative visions.

To be a creative woman, you must know your own value and regard your creative center as precious. Otherwise, you will easily forgo your feminine expression, desires, intuition, and other creative realms. Without self-value, you lose touch with your essential nature. Your wild feminine aches in response, and your root voice of sadness can guide you to the source of these losses. Whenever you discover a sense of sadness relating to your feminine self, you must spend time near the place of your loss. In doing so, you remember and lay claim to the forgotten regions of your creative range. Reflections about the root voice of sadness include:

Where do you have sadness or unresolved loss?

How do you protect yourself from feeling this hurt?

Where is your feminine potential waiting to be recognized?

### Women's Stories: Moving from Protection to Connection

During her pregnancy, Angela came to see me for relief from a sense of pelvic heaviness. While working on her body, I noticed a tremendous heaviness in her energy as well, which is often an emotional burden that a woman is carrying. I was also aware of the warmth emanating from Angela's center: the energy of her baby. Any blockages in a woman's energy system, such as pent-up emotional energy, take a toll on her body and limit her capacity for receiving the joy in her center. Emotional burdens that are carried in the female body, rather than expressed, always restrict a woman's energy flow and access to spirit in her root.

We completed the bodywork session, and I asked Angela how she had been doing. She replied that she had been feeling unexplainably sad. She was worried; she did not want her baby to be affected by her emotional state, and so she had tried to ignore her sadness. I shared my belief that Angela's baby was aware of her feelings because of their close proximity to one another.

Ignoring a feeling only increases its energetic load. And children, perhaps especially in utero, have a general sensitivity to their mother's emotional state. Although Angela wanted to protect her baby by holding back her feelings, it was more likely that this denial of emotion could register with her baby as a sign of disconnection. Acknowledging her emotional state did not mean that Angela would transfer her sadness to her baby. Instead, she could identify the needs contained within her emotions. The important thing was to stay aware of her root and connected with her baby while moving the energy of these feelings.

By sensing, rather than avoiding, her feelings, Angela would be showing her baby that emotions often relate to needs and that connection is an essential basis for healthy relationships. She could communicate with her baby (and later, her child) by saying, "I am feeling sad right now, and it does not have to do with you. I will be fine because my feelings help me understand what I want and need in my life, and from that, I learn how to take care of myself. Everyone feels sad sometimes, and even when I am sad I am still here for you." These statements would allow Angela's baby to feel safe in the knowledge that Angela was still available as a mother and that feelings can be a signal for self-care rather than simply carried as a burden. Many women attend to others and compromise their own self-care, yet everyone who has a personal relationship with a woman, as well as the woman herself, benefits when she attends to her core emotional health.

As we talked, I felt Angela's sadness dissipate and her baby settle. She told me at subsequent visits that she was feeling much better, and she realized that some of her sadness was related to the loss of freedom she anticipated in becoming a mother. When Angela acknowledged the feelings in her core, she was more aware of her negative associations with motherhood. Although paying attention to her emotional barometer made her more conscious of her perceptions about the limitations of motherhood, she also felt freer to challenge these perceived limitations. Emotions often direct a woman to areas that need attention in her creative life. Working with emotions, by clearing the energy and attending to the underlying needs, frees a woman's creative energy to be used in the manner she truly desires.

## A Call for Reconnection
When you hear your root voice of sadness, look for a place of disconnection. Listen to your feelings and recover the feminine

potential you contained before the losses that restricted your feminine range. Rather than avoiding your sadness, see how it leads you to forgotten parts of your inner wisdom, latent desires, creative dreams, or full relationship with spirit. Sadness calls you to find reconnection. You retrieve what holds value and meaning for you as a woman, finding your own expression of the feminine in the process. Reflections about sadness include:

How does your sadness call to you?
Which feminine realms will renew your creative connection and flow?

## Reveal Your Radiance

Women often dim their own radiance and limit the nourishment they are able to receive from their creative fire. Use the following exercise to identify these blocks that, when transformed, will reveal your radiance.

### Exercise: Reveal Your Radiance

1. On a piece of paper, list any blocks you may have about receiving the nourishment of your fire. For example: low self-value, limited time, unawareness of needs, busy taking care of others, distracted, and so on.

2. List any blocks to expressing your fire and revealing your radiance. For example: seems unsafe, will not be valued or acknowledged, not allowed to take up space, value linked to ability to produce, and so on.

3. Write three actions that encourage you to sit in the light of your fire. Place this list in a prominent place as a reminder for how to tend your creative flame.

# Cultivate the Fire in Your Belly

Sitting in a sweat lodge with five other women on the night of a new moon, it is dark. My eyes are open, but I see nothing. I forget about my eyes and notice instead the velvet earth, my wet skin, the breathing of women, the pine-smoke air. Without my eyes, I am more aware of my animal body, the fire in my belly. Fire-warmed rocks heat the inside of this earthen womb. I remember the fire in my mother's womb and the fire in my grandmothers'. I sit with five other women in the darkness. Only there is light, a fire in every woman's body, the fire of her creation.

## Ovarian Fire

Every woman can find ovarian balance and partake of the riches it bestows if she is willing to do the necessary work. It is critical to prune away any project that feels draining or is done from duty rather than desire. A woman must refuse any undertaking that does not inspire her (or feed her fire). If she uses her creative energy out of duty, even if the ventures themselves are well-intended, there is always a cost to her health. But if a woman follows her passions and interests, she runs her creative energy effortlessly. If she feels joy, she is using her energy in a sustainable manner—being nourished by the exchange, even as she gives of herself. Anything else is a drain on her energy that depletes her over time. When a woman finds ways to give that come from a place of joy, then this is her best offering.

We long to be fulfilled. To access our capacity for fulfillment, we need a robust left ovary—our link to the feminine—in our daily lives. Instead of looking to the outer world for validation, which is often fleeting at best, attuning to the feminine receptive nature will bring in the essence that feeds us. In the presence of the feminine, we become aware of the tangible beauty—the color of light, the touch of someone we love, the scent of flowers in bloom, the rustle of spirit moving nearby—that fills our bodies with energy. Then we can move into the right ovary, our masculine fire, with this fullness, rather than deficit, infusing our creation. We receive before we give, as part of the deep creative flow, and our creative lives reflect this sustainable pattern. Tending the home or giving of ourselves is joyful when we are being fed in the process.

Another way to work on ovarian balance is to do a daily gesture that draws on the energy of each ovary. In this way, you ensure nourishment for yourself and an outlet for your expression.

### Exercise: Daily Gestures for the Left and Right Ovaries

| Left Ovary | Right Ovary |
| --- | --- |
| Meditate on your pelvic bowl | Plan a women's gathering |
| Take a leisurely walk | Exercise |
| Read an inspirational book | Hone a new skill |
| Write in your journal | Share a creation with a friend |
| Soak in the bath | Volunteer where you feel inspired |
| Play with your clothes | Clean your closets |
| Take a nap | Find a new place to explore |
| Sip a cup of tea | Invite someone out for coffee |
| Make a nourishing soup | Try a new recipe |
| Look at your photo albums | Rearrange a room |
| Lie in the sun | Plant some seeds |
| Daydream | Take action on one of your dreams |

I have found that women have a tendency toward one ovary or the other, experiencing more comfort either with *doing* (right ovary activities) or *being* (left ovary activities). In the classes I teach, I ask women to meditate on their ovaries and then share which ovary was easier for them to connect with. Often the women who seem more outgoing and describe themselves as action-oriented connect to the right ovary. Similarly, the women who seem more internal and describe themselves as feeling-oriented connect to the left ovary. I imagine women someday describing themselves as a "left-ovary" or "right-ovary" type of woman. Indeed, we originate as an egg from only one of our mother's ovaries.

Still, it is beneficial to access both ovarian energies and to have them working together to shape our creations. In fact, the more that women use the energy of both the left and right ovaries, the greater the bridge will be between the inner and outer creative fires that will forge feminine values and principles into the external structures of our world.

A woman may also cultivate her creative fire by working directly with the energy of the ovaries. Directing breath to the ovaries is a powerful way to enliven their energy. The following breathing exercise has been used in my practice to assist women in developing their ovarian energy, and during it, women have reported an increased ability to feel their ovaries, while I have observed significant changes in their pelvic skin temperature, muscle tone, and overall ovarian energetic balance.

### Exercise: Gathering Ovarian Energy

Read the exercise through first, and then close your eyes to begin. Choose a comfortable position sitting or lying down.

1. Guide your attention to your pelvic bowl and be aware of any sensations that arise. Then bring your focus to the left ovary, felt as a warmth in the left side of your pelvis. Inhale and notice how the warmth of this fire might relate to your feminine radiance. As you exhale, breathe slowly into this ovary as if blowing on a hot coal. Now inhale and invite the left ovary to expand its energy into your left pelvis by spreading its warmth in a greater space. Allow it to nourish your left breast. Repeat this cycle three to five times.

2. Shift your focus to your right ovary, in the same location on the opposite side of your pelvis. Inhale and notice how the warmth of this fire might relate to your masculine radiance. Slowly exhale, blowing into your right ovary. Then inhale and invite the right ovary to expand its energy into your right pelvis. Allow it to nourish your right breast. Repeat this cycle three to five times.

3. If either ovary has a diffuse sensation or unclear edges, simply guide your awareness around the edge of your pelvis and imagine scooping the ovary's energy back toward its center.

4. Continue with three to five breath cycles, directing your exhale to both ovaries simultaneously. Let the heat of your ovaries warm and revitalize your whole pelvic bowl. Ponder the transformative power of fire: burning wood to ash, boiling water for cooking food, melting rock into metal. Your body contains this transformative potential.

5. Notice your pelvic bowl again. Do you have more awareness or a greater sensation of warmth in the pelvic space around your ovaries? How is the radiance of your feminine and masculine fire? After completing this exercise, compare the sensations of your left and right ovaries and the balance in your core. Give thanks to the ovaries and the fire in your bowl.

**Transform Ovarian Energetic Patterns**
Whether you seek to open a blockage or restore conscious awareness, transforming ovarian energetic patterns involves bringing your full presence to each ovary. Use the previous exercise to gather your ovarian energy and strengthen it. Pay attention daily

to changes. The energy flow of the ovaries often stops abruptly in the midst of stress or with a disruption in the energy field caused by a disturbing situation or event. Learning to sense the subtle shifts in the core of your body can alert you to patterns of unintentionally shutting down your core energy flow. After noticing an ovarian pattern of disconnection or blockage in a specific situation, restore a normal energy flow to your ovaries with focused breathing, and you will also restore the vibrant and protective nature of your pelvic energy field.

As you transition to a place of greater energetic balance, you may notice that your ovaries reveal different imbalances in various aspects of your life or as you heal from events associated with the past. This may occur as you travel back through previous layers of energy held in your core. Notice these shifts and continue the process of reclaiming and reviving the energy of these vital feminine organs.

When you begin to change the energetic patterns of your ovaries, you may feel an ache or twinge in your right or left pelvis. This sensation occurs as a greater energy flow returns. Pay attention to what is taking place in your life when you experience these ovarian sensations. Try to determine what your body may be calling attention to. Then place your hands over your ovaries, use focused breathing to gather your ovarian energy, soften your lower belly, and increase the warmth and energy flow in your pelvis. Particularly when you feel upset, check your inner sensation of ovarian energy flow to see if you have reverted to a pattern of imbalance. Practice working with your ovaries so that in times of stress you can reactivate their energy as a source of support.

Transforming a blocked left ovary pattern allows the stagnant energy to move so that you can expand beyond a limited notion of female identity and receive your full feminine range. You can then choose what energy and creative impulses you bring into your body and daily life. Accessing the left ovary invites the playful aspects of your feminine spirit to inspire and delight you. This lighthearted essence is the energy that propels your soul's work.

Likewise, opening a blocked right ovary invites expanding beyond the culturally defined limitations for the expressions of your creative power. It brings your own personal relationship with the feminine into being to create new masculine forms and modes of living. It guards your creative potential for use in your own life. Your right ovarian energy helps change family and cultural patterns conflicting with your feminine spirit; it is essential for embodying the full vibrancy of your creative life.

Restoring consciousness to an absent or overactive ovary means examining beliefs or habits that feed off these energetic imbalances. Begin by noticing patterns such as letting others define your femininity, blocking your self-nurturance, or giving away your creative power. When you become conscious of these patterns, you will be able to change your ovarian receptive and projective abilities.

### Exercise: Cultivating Ovarian Energy Flow

Reflect on your patterns of creative energy usage with this exercise.

1. Reflection: Notice how your creative energy is both received and expressed in your life. What nourishment do you take in on a regular basis? How are you using your creative essence outwardly? Ponder the role of your ovarian energy in your creative ventures, your feminine-masculine flow, and making a joy-filled life. Refuel your fire by bringing in more nourishment or giving yourself another form of expression.

2. Ritual: Ponder a creative inspiration that you want to give more attention to. Ask your left ovary what is needed to nurture this inspiration. Ask your right ovary how to give form

to this inspiration in your life. Honor the fire of your ovaries and you will enliven their creative flow.

As you cultivate the fire of your ovaries, observe the wisdom they offer. Your left ovary will teach you about receiving and nourishing your feminine spirit. Your right ovary will lead you to the creative abundance you desire. As catalysts in creative projects, intimate relationships, and other passionate sparks, the ovaries deserve your care and attention.

## Fallopian Tubes: Sustain Your Partnerships

The opposing play of ovarian and uterine energies creates a purposeful tension. The uterus has a more serious nature than the ovaries, as fits her tasks. These tasks may include holding and nourishing a baby as well as containing the focused and determined energy behind any project a woman takes on. The ovaries keep energy moving and inspired, reminding the uterus to find time to play, even as she does her hard work. The fallopian tubes sustain the connection between them.

As the connection between the ovaries and uterus, the fallopian tubes symbolize the health of your creative partnerships. They provide a vital link between the opposing energetic forces of your fiery ovarian energy and steadfast uterine energy. While the energetic relationship between the ovaries and uterus is not always an easy one, it enables you to cultivate your creative fire in a sustainable manner. Reflections on the fallopian tubes include:

How do you coordinate the relationship between receiving creative inspiration and doing the work of manifesting your creations?

Where are you challenged by the opposing nature of this creative tension?

What partnerships would you like to change or develop to support your creative work?

### Exercise: Nurturing Your Creative Partnerships

This exercise will enhance your ability to create and build connections between your different sources of feminine creative energy. Read through the exercise first, and then close your eyes to begin. Find a comfortable position sitting or lying down.

1. Guide your attention internally to your pelvic space and notice any sensations that arise. Notice the relationship between each ovary and your uterus. Try to visualize as well as sense the energetic and physical fallopian tube connection on your right and left sides.

2. If one connection feels blocked or difficult to access, send your breath along a path from your ovary to the uterus. Visualize an ovum or light moving along this path as it follows your breath.

3. Focus on the right fallopian tube if you are presently cultivating external work or partnerships. Focus on the left fallopian tube if you are refining your relationship to the feminine or other creative connections. Repeat five to seven breath cycles.

4. Ask your uterus and ovaries if anything is needed to enhance their partnership.

5. Offer gratitude to your fallopian tubes for providing their crucial link and notice any changes in the sensations of your pelvic space.

## Fallopian Tube Disconnections

As the meeting place between a woman's ovarian creative potential and uterine place of gestation, the fallopian tubes are frequently a place of energetic disconnection when a woman represses her creative essence.

### Women's Stories: Remembering Her Authentic Beauty

Marissa experienced cramping with ovulation—especially when she ovulated on the left side—that seemed to increase as she approached perimenopause. Energy imbalances and tension in the pelvis can increase sensations of cramping with both ovulation and menstruation. I guided Marissa's attention to her pelvic space and began to instruct her in an ovarian breathing exercise. After a few cycles of breathing, she visualized her right ovary as a bright ball of light. In contrast, her left ovary appeared dark and withered. She described her left ovary as "off by itself and far way from the rest of her womb." She also held more tension on the left side of her pelvic bowl.

I guided her in an exercise that focused her breath and attention on the left fallopian tube, the connection between the left ovary and uterus. While doing this, Marissa had a sudden thought—she remembered a time as a young woman when she was just discovering her own sense of style. Initially, trying on makeup and clothing felt like an anticipated rite of passage. Looking for inspiration, she sought and began to imitate the styles in beauty magazines. At first, she felt confident in her own way of being, but the mainstream beauty images and messages began to dominate her self-expression.

The more Marissa compared and tried to conform to an external version of beauty, the more she judged herself. She felt a growing feeling of inadequacy just as she was beginning to discover her budding womanhood. Rather than continue to explore her own expression, she internalized a narrowly defined vision of femininity and unconsciously restricted her creative range. Rejecting the part of herself that yearned to express her beauty, she gave up this aspect of her feminine ground.

More recently, Marissa found herself continuously frustrated in her relationships with men, and by focusing on the root of her body, she discovered the source. She longed to experience her femininity in a beautiful, sensual way. Yet, instead of creating her own expression, Marissa relied on men to make her feel beautiful. She realized that her self-prescribed beauty routine and rigorous exercise program had become regimens that felt constraining, reinforcing a restrictive and often unattainable sense of beauty. Her earlier negative imprint had caused her to diminish her feminine energy, and Marissa's left ovary and access to her feminine sensuality had been long forgotten. As she remembered her initial playful response to her own radiance, she rediscovered a desire for authentic feminine expression.

When a woman's outer creativity or sense of her own ability to create value or beauty is restricted, it blocks the natural energy flow in the pelvic space. Over time, this blockage causes pelvic tension and other physical imbalances. Core tension and pelvic imbalance can make ovulation or menstruation painful, when each has the potential to be a pleasurable sense of release.

Doing her own vaginal self-massage over the next several weeks, Marissa released the tension in her core and listened to the true desires of her body. She also used her breath and internal awareness to reconnect the energies of her uterus (her core womanhood) and her left ovary (her forgotten feminine range). Reconnecting with the feminine part of herself, Marissa was inspired to actively express her beauty rather than rely on a partner to fulfill her feminine needs. She acknowledged her body's desire to express her own style, eat more fresh food, and go out dancing. Receiving the energy of her left ovary, Marissa would nourish her body and make room for a robust expression of the feminine in her life.

## Manifest Your Creative Visions

The fallopian tubes are symbolic of the creative partnerships and tensions that enable a woman to manifest her creative visions. Notice your own patterns of initiating, cocreating, building, sustaining, and releasing creative ventures in order to understand the role this energy plays in your life.

### *Exercise: Fallopian Tube Energy Reflected in Your Life*

1. Reflection: Notice the essential partnerships or creative collaborations you have made. What connections have presently formed around your creations? Ponder how a break in partnership or a period of solitary creation has served your path. Reflect on any blockages in your ability to create with others or in the presence of dynamic creative tension.

2. Ritual: Make a plan to gather with some women friends to celebrate each of your newest creations. Honor the creative partnerships in your body and life for the way they sustain your creative visions.

## Gather with Other Women

Have you noticed the satisfaction in your body when you spend an evening in the company of other women? Your body, your wild feminine, craves this female connection. Make space for shared dinners, book groups, knitting circles, and other gatherings that celebrate feminine creativity. Whether casual or created with specific intention, these gatherings refuel your creative essence. Powerful things happen when women come together.

In my workshops, women sit with one another and the energy that is moved is greater than what one woman can make by herself. Many times, a woman has been struggling with an issue in her life, but when she brings it forward in the circle of women, it is no longer hers alone. She leaves the circle and discovers in the passing days and weeks that her struggle has changed. The energy has been transformed by the collective power of female energy.

Tend your creative fire as a woman. Seek the creative partnerships that enliven your potential, and expand your creative visions as directed by your wild feminine spirit. Notice the forms of feminine and masculine expression that draw you to others—whether through joint projects, ritual, food, or some other medium. Cultivate the fire in your belly and be warmed by the fire of your making.

*May you delight in the radiance that shines from within.*

# FIVE

# Returning to the Mother Place

*The womb is one of the wisest places in the female body and one of
the most ignored. Though we may listen to her in regard to birthing
babies, we ought to be listening in terms of our whole creative lives.
One of my teachers, Rosita Arvigo, relates a story from her teacher,
Don Elijio, a Maya healer born in the late 1800s. He spoke of his
village gathering around the fire in the morning to listen to the dreams
of the menstruating women for the psychic information they contained.
We need to remember our way back to this kind of knowing—that
the living energies of our bodies relate deeply to the movement of
our lives. This chapter examines the patterns of creative flow that
arise from the womb, the most powerful energy patterns for
building and sustaining a woman's creative life and dreams.*

With five small bowls that fit neatly together, one inside the
other, I am teaching women about the power of the uterus.
The largest bowl fits in the palm of my hand, and the smallest is
the size of a pencil eraser. These bowls represent the way that the
uterus holds energy and passes information from one generation to
another. The women watch my hands as I align the bowls, one by
one, according to their size.

I point to the smallest bowl, saying, "This is you." Slipping this
tiny bowl into the next one I say, "You were held in your mother's
womb." Placing the two bowls together into the next bowl I say,
"Your mother's eggs were fully formed while she was held in her
mother's body. In this way, you were also held in your grandmother's

womb." I continue to join the bowls together, until the five are sitting in my palm, one inside the other. "Because your grandmother carries the energy of her mother's and grandmother's wombs, so you are linked to them as well." The bowls rest neatly in my hand. The women sit squarely in front of me. I see each of them wrapped in layers of female energy from the women ancestors who came before them.

I set the bowls down. "Now, this is you," I tell them, pointing to the largest bowl. From the large bowl I lift the next bowl, which still holds three others. "This is one of your creations," I say. One by one, I lift the smaller bowls and place each next to the bowl that served as its container. With each bowl, I tell the women, "This is the seed of one of your creations." I continue until the five bowls, five generations, sit in a line. Each bowl is separate, but the action of lifting one bowl from the next illustrates their shared lineage, or line of descendants. "This is how your womb and the energy that you carry there influence all you create. The energy in your pelvic bowl is your mark on the future; this is your legacy of creation." The room is silent as the women remember their mother place.

## The Mother Place

The uterus is our direct connection to the sacred; the womb is a woman's place for co-creating with spirit and mothering her creations. I have sat with many women as they rediscovered the mother place in their bodies and I have witnessed the grief and joy they associate with their creative essence. Every woman has a place in herself to mother from, regardless of whether or not she has given birth to a child. But many women close the door to their womb if they are unable to own the word *mother*.

To understand our collective ambivalence about ourselves as mothers, we need to look at those who come to inhabit that role by having a child. For example, when women come to my office, they fill out intake forms with a variety of medical and personal information, including their occupation. Sometimes mothers, who remain in the home as the primary caretakers for their children, but have no official work title, scoff at the notion of occupation and question what they could possibly write in that space. I was initially taken aback by this, and I have spent time thinking about why women who are mothers hesitate to claim the word/identity *mother*. Clearly, the predominant culture has not placed value on the role of mother. Still, each of these clients is keenly aware of how much they do each day in the name of motherhood. Each cherishes her child and their relationship. Yet, when putting pen to paper, *mother* is still not enough. In our reactions to the notion of mother, we see the work that remains to be done to reclaim the true essence of mothering.

Until women themselves value and honor mothering in all its forms, there is little chance that the cultural paradigms will change. Many women with children have come to respect the art of mothering, but they still need to internalize its value in order to be able to advocate for their needs when faced with external expectations and pressures to feel professional success. Likewise, mothers who work outside the home must hold their professional and mothering roles in equal measure. Mothering is a profoundly spiritual and creative process, yet remains unclaimed as such. I attended a women's celebration where the female speakers listed their vocations: storyteller, healer, doctor, lawyer, teacher, musician, artist, and so on. Many of them were mothers, but the word *mother* never appeared.

I have often found that women who have not given birth or raised children typically disown their mothering capacity altogether. Some of these women hold unprocessed grief from a sense of unrealized potential, yet working with the grief in their center will ultimately restore full connection to their creative essence. Other women have chosen to direct their creative energies into other capacities besides having children, but typically still have deep conflicts about their mothering essence that will remain unresolved unless addressed with intention. For each woman, it is essential to recognize that her body craves the creative flow and sense of her soul unfolding that comes from working with this internal mothering capacity.

Women want to be valued for all aspects of our feminine selves and to live in ways that encourage us to nourish ourselves and the home fire, whether or not we have children. To accomplish this, we must reclaim the power of the word mother, and every woman must negotiate this mother-place terrain in order to fully cherish her creative essence. Unless she learns to celebrate her own potential for mothering, a woman will compromise her ability to gestate or sustain creations, perhaps settling for less than she truly is capable of creating.

### Women's Stories: Reclaiming Her Mothering Energy

When Sandra came to my office, she had the makings of a happy life. She had her own successful design business, a fulfilling partnership, and many friends. She had consciously chosen not to have children, but internally, she also felt that something was missing. I spent some time evaluating her pelvis and noticed that her uterine energy was low. When I shared my surprise at finding low uterine energy, because she was clearly using her creative abilities in starting a business and working in the field of design, Sandra replied that she was really a painter, but because of the demands of her business, she found little time for painting.

I directed her to focus on her womb and pay attention to what she was presently gestating there. She closed her eyes and thought for a moment. When she opened them, she said she saw an image of her mother. Sandra explained that her mother was an alcoholic, emotionally dysfunctional, and virtually unable to provide any mothering. For as long as she could remember, Sandra had taken care of her mother. Since she had so many projects at work, she thought her own creative energy would be taken up with one of them. But beneath her busy life, she found that her uterine energy was still maintaining an old family pattern of caretaking.

Sandra's situation is not uncommon—many children step in to parent a family member. While this may have been necessary at one time, continuing to energetically take care of her mother was draining Sandra's creative vitality. Just becoming aware of this pattern in her pelvic space was an essential first step to reclaiming her creative energy for herself.

As Sandra breathed deeply into her core, she pondered her choice to remain childless. Perhaps she had never wanted children because mothering felt like such a burden and she had expended her creative essence primarily on taking care of the overwhelming needs of her mother. Now, feeling her womb for herself, Sandra could see the potential she contained for creating whatever she wanted. She was inspired to gather her paints and start a fresh canvas.

A woman's creative potential is easily co-opted if she does not recognize and cultivate it as her own. Use the following exercise to examine your relationship to the word mother and the way you relate to your creative ground.

### Exercise: Redefining Mother

1. On a piece of paper, draw a circle. Inside of the circle, write all the positive associations that come to mind when you think about the word *mother*.

2. Outside of the circle, write any negative associations that come to mind when reflecting on *mother*.

3. Though both positive and negative words may relate to your mothering identity, think of the circle as your pelvic bowl and symbolic of your power to hold what you chose. The way that you conceive of *mother* defines how you relate to or reject your creative essence and affects how you inhabit or disown your mother place.

4. Reflect on your positive associations. How do you connect with these attributes on a daily basis? Choose three to work with and make note of a specific action that will encourage these qualities in your body and creative life.

5. Reflect on your negative associations. In what ways do these words call for a healing action? Choose three to work with and make note of a specific action that overcomes these limitations, allowing you to further reclaim your mothering ground.

6. Ponder all the mothers and other creative women you know. Let the diversity of these women inspire you to expand and further redefine your own mothering form. Give thanks for the mothers and the place of mothering in your life.

## Uterine Energy and Your Feminine Power

Living in a household of males, I have come to know the power of my uterus. Whenever I am in the house, my sons find me and circle round like satellites. It is not that they look for me; rather, their bodies draw them intuitively to my side. Many times, I have sought a quiet corner, away from the high-energy cluster, only to find that, within minutes, my sons, and often my husband, seek me out.

Male and female bodies process energy distinctly. Though there is individual variation, generally the female body takes energy in, transforms, and then releases this energy. The male body projects energy outward, propelling him to the receptor of his energy. Tending to my young sons, I have noticed their continuous desires to throw, push, and pound. As my sons run and wrestle, they express their male need to externalize energy. Likewise, my feminine ability to hold and gestate energy frequently calls them to me.

## Recognize Your Feminine Power

In the uterus, the center of the pelvic bowl, lies the feminine power to create. This includes two aspects: receptivity and release. The receptive potential of the uterus, which receives, holds, and transforms energy in the female body, is most easily seen in the process of pregnancy. The releasing potential of the uterus, with energy propelled outward, is most obviously witnessed in the birth of a child. Whether a woman is making children or other works of the womb, the creative power of her uterus is amazing to behold. Some of a woman's most profound transformations involve the changes in her womb: menarche, pregnancy, miscarriage, childbirth, and menopause.

Every womb desires to give birth by receiving and gestating a particular energy; yet the way a woman specifically utilizes her creative energy is a matter of personal intention. One woman may use the energetic capacity for creation in her work as an artist or other creative endeavor. Another woman relies on her creative energy to nurture her children or reinvent her mothering. A spiritual teacher may receive a divine energy, gestating rituals for celebrating the sacred. A healer uses her intuitive capacity to aid others in physical, energetic, and emotional transformation.

### Exercise: Creative Essence Meditation

Imagine your creative essence, your mothering energy. Pay attention to what it looks like or how it feels.

1. Reflection: Now bring awareness to your womb space. Ponder how you are presently using your female energy to create

or sustain aspects of your life. Is this how you want to use your creative essence? Is there anything else that calls to you? Are you nourishing yourself as part of your creative process?

2. Ritual: Find a place to sit where you are directly in contact with the earth. Let the mothering energy of your womb arise from the seasonal energy of the earth. Feel the sustenance of the earth replenishing your womb. How will this energy flow impact the design of your creations? Think of a simple image or action that will remind you to connect with and create from this daily flow in your core.

## Uterine Energy

The uterus holds or releases energy, moving through the cycle of transformation, in relationship to the womb's reproductive cycle. Held uterine energy is created when a woman is pregnant or while building a menstrual lining, and sustains a period of gestation for the uterus and female body. In contrast, released uterine energy is created during events such as birth and menstruation. At these times the uterus has a physical and energetic release to cleanse and rejuvenate a woman's pelvis and to bring her creations into being. If a woman is no longer menstruating, her body still has internal creative cycles that may relate to the moon cycle (a full moon corresponding to uterine held energy and a new moon to uterine release) or other life cycle. Accessing the full range of uterine energy allows a woman to consciously cultivate her core energy and follow her inner creative rhythm. *Note*: Even after a hysterectomy, a woman can cultivate the creative center related to the womb.

## Held Uterine Energy: A Period of Gestation

A woman experiences held uterine energy during a period of gestation or preparation for new life. This energy has a feeling of fullness, like ripe summer fruit, as energy moves into the womb to sustain a woman's creations. Uterine energy is vigorous and robust whether it is used for gestating a child or for other creative ventures. Held energy provides nourishment during the creative process and protects creations that are still developing. Reflections on held uterine energy include:

What are you presently holding or gestating in your life?
What would you like to gather or hold in your life as a woman?
What is needed to make space for creating what you want?

### Exercise: Holding Your Creations

When your womb is full, in the mode of gestation, receive your womb wisdom by using this meditation.

1. Close your eyes and bring awareness to your womb space.

2. Feel the energy in your womb. Notice your creative center. What are you presently gestating? How does this reflect your creative dreams? What will support this gestation?

3. Look to the front of your pelvic bowl. Take a breath in and direct it to the front of your bowl. Think about giving form to this creation. Acknowledge any fears or hesitations you may have. Surround your creative core with your breath, allowing your energy to move and open any restrictions. Let yourself be further inspired, even by limitations that you may encounter.

4. Look to the back of your pelvic bowl. Reflect on the path that led you to this creative moment. Acknowledge the work you have done and the assistance received on this creative

journey. Is there additional support you need for yourself or this creation?

5. Set your intention for the approaching birth or unveiling of your creation. What assistance will you need from others? What do you desire for yourself and this creation in the outer world? How will you celebrate and continue to be nourished by this creation?

6. Offer gratitude for your abundance and for those who have provided for you on this creative journey.

## Uterine Energy Release: A Time of Letting Go

Released uterine energy pertains to death or the release of life. Many people in Western culture have an aversion to the word *death* and avoid acknowledging its inevitability. However, as a cyclical aspect of transformation, death ultimately enhances life. Seasonal death, like wintertime, is the energetic movement of surrender, a natural dying back that serves as a renewal before life begins again.

The uterus releases energy during a woman's bleeding time and anytime she consciously makes a ritual or retreat for herself. Embracing a period of release allows a woman to shed self-limiting beliefs and extraneous energy to reveal her authentic nature and emphasize what is truly essential in her life. When the female body begins to release, a woman may feel vulnerable because her energy field is more diffuse, as if her cells have spread apart to allow a release of energy from deep within her core. This vulnerability invites a woman to be more internal and solitary so that, rather than distracted by outer demands, she can receive intuitive information and do the work of her own energetic house cleaning.

Each uterine release allows a woman to grow and evolve her core patterns. She emerges from her retreat, prepared for the next creative cycle. Dissolving old forms and identities, released uterine energy propels a woman through periods of transformation and brings her to a new way of being. Support a release with an exercise for clearing the womb space (page 220). Reflections about uterine energy release include:

What are you presently releasing from your life?
What else would you like to release or let go of?
What is needed for you to fully surrender these things?

Finding power in the root of your female body means knowing what you want to hold or release from your pelvic bowl. You have more choice about how to use your creative energy when your pelvic bowl is clear.

## Grief: Lighten Your Load

Initially, I was surprised by the depth of grief I encountered while working in the root of the female body. As I came to understand the capacity of the female body for holding energy, particularly the energy of unrecognized events and feelings, these vast reservoirs of grief made sense. Unless there are rituals or other means to channel the energy of grief, it sits like a stone in a woman's pelvis.

From the degree of unaddressed emotions I encounter in the pelvic space, I know that women are presently carrying much grief on behalf of their families. This is particularly true because, in general, Western culture lacks rituals for acknowledging and releasing the energy of grief. As the energy keeper in a family, a woman holds the energy of those around her; a woman's bodily grief, potentially arising from many individuals—not just herself—becomes a burden. Without the ritual or collective acknowledgment and release of grief, women carry that energy. Any unexpressed emotional energy requires a woman to hold tension in her body, which interferes with her ability to be at ease in her core.

A collection of unexpressed grief decreases a woman's presence in her root, limiting her creative expression and capacity for intimate relationships. A woman's own radiance is dimmed by the energy required to maintain a storehouse of grief. After witnessing the change in a woman's pelvis, energetically and physically, when she releases this stored grief, I have seen the potential that lies in relinquishing this weight.

It is surprising and delightful that when grief held in the female body is acknowledged, it begins to move out of a woman's core. The heavy sensation of held grief lifts. When the womb is lighter, a woman's creative center is available to mother her own creations. When a woman attends to her grief, she discovers where to lighten her load.

## The Importance of Grief Rituals

For centuries women have performed grief rituals to acknowledge and clear community grief. A memorial is an example of a grief ritual for the death of an individual. However, without regular release through community grief rituals, most grief remains unmourned, its energy trapped and burdensome.

In an effort to address my own grief and transform the lineage that I pass to my children, I made a grief ritual for my family. When we gathered for this ritual, we covered a long stick with strips of paper holding the words of our grief. Then, to symbolically release our grief, we threw this stick into the great Columbia River.

As my brother and son tossed our grief-laden stick high into the air, a single piece of paper fell away. We gasped as it floated nearby. With so many papers tied on and layered over one another, only one message of grief had fallen from the bundle. I snatched it up, wondering whose it could be, only to recognize my own handwriting. I laughed out loud, faced with my own grief.

Quickly, I tied my grief paper to another stick and threw it out again. Still unsatisfied with where it had landed, I plunged into the water. I plucked out my grief and hurled it into the air. My family cheered as my lone stick caught up to and sailed past our group stick. "Ha ha," I called to this grief, feeling victorious and relieved all at once.

"Imagine the river full of sticks like ours, all of the grief being acknowledged and released," said one person. We watched our grief float away until there was nothing more to see. My uterus ached as if I had given birth. I had released the energy of my grief. That night, I dreamed I was back in the river, giving birth to a white ball of light. I set this light into the water and heard the voices of women singing. I awoke with these words in my head: *Now I too can sing*.

Grief is a natural and purposeful response to any life-changing event. When it is allowed its expression, it brings a liminal or altered state that reorients a woman's path, inviting her to go deeper within herself. What was known previously is no longer true. The grief process strips away the extraneous—energetic and otherwise. Moving her bodily grief ultimately facilitates the creation of new beliefs and structures that will better assist a woman on her life journey.

My family's grief ritual is outlined below. Some women I have worked with have made their own variations. While this ritual is simple, when grief is intentionally acknowledged the resulting lightness of spirit is quite profound.

### *Exercise: Creating a Grief Ritual*

1. Invitation: Explain to friends and/or family that you are gathering a group together with the shared intention of releasing the burden of grief. Invite them to reflect inwardly, without speaking, on the grief they carry, both as individuals and as a part of their lineage.

2. Preparation: Explain that each person will write on separate pieces of paper any words relating to grief that come to mind. Then the pieces of paper will be tied to a stick that will either

be burned or thrown into a river, as you choose. Distribute paper, pens, and string.

3. Inspiration: Each person writes for as long as needed. Those who have finished fold and tie their paper onto the stick.

4. Celebration: Choose someone to throw the stick into the fire or water while everyone else claps, chants, cheers, observes, or does what they are moved to do.

5. Restoration: Come back to the circle and share observations with one another. On one piece of paper, write words of hope or prayers that can be taken home and placed on an altar or buried in the earth of your yard, wherever beauty is cultivated. If time permits, have a meal together and inwardly note any changes within yourself, in the sensations of your body, or the sense of your community.

## The Root Voice of Grief: Burdens of Womanhood

Women share a collective sense of grief based on the history of being repressed rather than being held in high regard, for not being celebrated as females. This voice speaks of sexual abuse and other violations of the female body and feminine spirit. It speaks of ill-defined femininity, held in place by men and women who have embodied the distortion that limits women's (and men's) full expression, derides deviations from prescribed roles, and continues to degrade the feminine.

Women also grieve personally for the losses experienced in life's inevitable transitions. The changes in identity that occur as a woman moves through different phases and roles are accompanied by this sense of grief, even when she welcomes these shifts in her life. If she delves into her feminine grief on these occasions, she will be richer for the experience.

Knowing that grief held in the womb is somewhat universal helps to prepare a woman to encounter her own. A colleague described her midwifery training, when she and her classmates practiced pelvic exams on one another; the palpable grief made the air in the room unbearably heavy and dense as they approached the sadness in each other's wombs. Yet grief is purposeful when it is acknowledged and released.

One of the most profound places of pelvic or uterine grief is a lost pregnancy, which may be carried with a woman all her life, unraveling over time. I have seen a woman grieve for a pregnancy that occurred twenty years previously, the cold sensation of death still hovering in her womb until she was finally able to work directly with the energy of this loss.

The event of a soul passing on within her body touches each woman in a different way. Yet it also links her to a broader community of women who share in the transformative effects of such grief. When a spirit touches down in a woman's womb and leaves from this place as well, a woman experiences the entry and exit of a soul within her body. When a whole life is contained within the womb without coming to term, a powerful invitation is given to the mother—to connect with the spiritual realm in the core of her body, to sit with her grief and come to know the spirit of her child.

When a woman loses a baby in the later stages of pregnancy, it is more common for her to mourn this loss. But no matter how long a woman carries a baby, this life asks to be acknowledged and remembered, witnessed and loved. The energy that comes in with each life still must be moved. Without the natural movement of energy that occurs with a typical birth, a woman may have to be more conscious about working with the energy in her core. But if she receives the energy of this soul into her womb and then gives it an expression in her outer life, then she also receives a blessing.

My own pregnancy loss by miscarriage was a profound event in my body and my life. The spirit who came to be with me brought tremendous healing and creative energy to my womb that continues to inspire me today. If you have experienced a womb loss, you can still celebrate this soul's life. For example, you can plant a tree to acknowledge what you experienced or learned as a witness. Ask your body how else you might remember the essence of this spirit.

Work with the grief you encounter in your pelvic bowl, whether through ritual, art, intimate conversation, or some other mode of expression. Felt grief will liberate your female energy; instead of merely holding back the tide of grief, your creative essence is free to actively inspire your creations. Reflections on grief include:

What losses are expressed by your root voice of grief?
If you have been touched by a womb loss, what did you
　　witness in the life and passing of this soul?
How will you remember this soul's essence?

In calling to mind your grief, feel the energetic weight that it contains. When you pay attention to the sensations or qualities of this energy, your sense of this grief will begin to change. Initially, you will feel the heaviness of grief gradually lift as its wave-like movements wash over you. If you continue to witness your grief, you will emerge with the clarity and lightness that is typical of felt grief. It is a restorative process that ultimately prepares you for new ground.

### Exercise: Marking Your Grief

1. Reflection: Take a moment to reflect on your grief. Ponder your held grief by responding to the following statement: "I have grief for ..." Pay attention to whatever comes to mind. Write without stopping for ten minutes, or longer if you like.

2. Ritual: Take the piece of paper containing your grief and plant it in the earth as a symbol of setting down burdens of grief. Say: "I lay my grief to rest." The earth can hold and transform this grief as nourishment for something else to grow; it no longer needs to be carried. Create a community grief ritual (with one or more people) for any grief that persists.

## Own Your Pelvic Bowl

The pelvic bowl belongs to each woman, but to claim it you must discover what is held in your center. You may hold the memory of a particular wound or painful experience that went unrecognized. You may encounter emotions that were left unexpressed for yourself or others you have cared for. When the pelvic bowl contains unacknowledged pain or emotional burdens, it depletes your creative energy. It is a place to cultivate feminine vitality, not a storehouse for past hurts.

Bring awareness to your root and notice what is here for you. Acknowledge the feelings and experiences of your womanhood that call for your attention. Clear the grief or other feelings you carry for those who could not contain their own emotions. You are the rightful keeper of your pelvic bowl.

*Women's Stories: Processing the Grief for Her Family's Losses*

Sally had a miscarriage, and she came for pelvic work to support her post-miscarriage healing. The physical and energetic pelvic structure after miscarriage is similar to that of a woman postpartum because the uterus has opened and birthed. While it does not have to dilate as fully as with a full-term birth, the uterus also does not have enough time to process the rapid pace of conception, birth, and loss that occurs in a miscarriage.

As we began vaginal massage and pelvic breathing exercises to restore Sally's pelvic balance, she immediately encountered a powerful sense of grief. First, she found her own grief at losing this child. Next, she saw an image of her uterus crying and rocking back and forth. This surprised Sally, to find that her body itself might also grieve a miscarriage.

Then Sally found another voice of grief—it was the voice of her husband, Mark. She thought about his experience of grieving this miscarriage. Mark was calm whenever Sally was crying or feeling grief but became irritable between these moments of her grief. Because he rarely cried, Sally surmised that she was processing the grief for their family.

Sally also remembered that her mother previously had a miscarriage, just before her pregnancy with Sally. After recognizing their common thread of grief, Sally returned home and called her mother. In their conversation, Sally learned that her mother had never thought to acknowledge her own miscarriage loss because she was encouraged to just "move on." Still mourning her own loss, Sally now found herself tapping into another source of sadness: the held grief within her of her mother's unmourned miscarriage. The grief of Sally's father had also gone unacknowledged, because in those days, men were not considered to be involved until after a baby's birth. But both partners experience grief with a miscarriage. When these feelings are unexpressed, they remain near the place of loss, in this case the womb where Sally was later conceived.

After speaking with her mother, Sally lit two candles, one for each of their baby's spirits. She mourned for both of them, and for the many times she had felt alone while experiencing a loss. She found that acknowledging these losses deepened her sense of connection with her mother, through their shared womb events. Moving the grief energy, she also felt a quiet inner peace that brought healing and a sacred connection to her baby. Witnessing her husband and thinking about her father, Sally felt compassion for the ways men are discouraged from expressing their grief or receiving comfort.

When Sally returned for her next session with me, she described feeling significantly lighter in her pelvic space. Learning about her mother's loss had enabled her to honor her own miscarriage and to find a more intimate connection with her mother. By attending to her pelvis and noticing how she felt in her center, she also knew when to encourage her husband to address his feelings about the loss of their baby. Sally's grief still arose at unexpected moments, but each wave of grief left a new sense of connection in its wake.

## Acknowledge What You Hold

Whether grief or other feelings you encounter in your womanhood are your own or held for someone else, they need to be acknowledged and released. Unacknowledged feelings become stagnant and bitter, resulting in patterns of self-blame, creating additional grief, and adding heft to your burden. Emotions that are witnessed will dissipate: your energy freed, your load lifted.

Notice any thoughts that limit your emotional expression or release. Allow your feelings to surface. Note thoughts that appear, such as: *I need to hold this grief so someone will love me* or *It is my responsibility to hold this pain.* If you are carrying the weight of emotions that reflect a profound loss but do not seem relevant to your present life, then you may be containing emotional energy for a parent, other caregiver, or even a distant member of your lineage. Children are often empathetic to their parents and caregivers, taking on their emotional burdens, hoping to lighten the energy in the home. Emotional family patterns may also be passed along to children as gender-based expectations (for example, all the women are angry or all the men are depressed). However, as an adult, you can change these patterns that influence your feminine and masculine energy and consciously choose what you hold in your bowl.

Working with profound grief and other emotions that you encounter in your root may require the assistance of others. When mourning a profound loss, it is difficult to overcome the emotional mixture of betrayal and grief on your own. Facing the unmet needs of your childhood self can be overwhelming and may trigger feelings of helplessness and despair. However, moving the energy of each loss imprinted in your root will invite you to find a deeper relationship with spirit and discover what is real and true for you. Listen to your root voice of grief to learn where to lighten your load and transform what you carry.

Intentionally releasing emotional burdens may inspire you to create a healing movement, such as a group ritual, an art piece, or an altar space. For example: Create a work of art while pondering the places that your radiance was restricted, and then examine the art and see what you learn. Create a second work of art that engages the restriction in a dynamic manner or expands beyond it so that you witness the potential to change these defining lines. Then invite other women to gather, share their own experience of this exercise, and celebrate their radiant selves. The process of creating in the presence of pain and engaging with the places where our creative essence has been blocked or dissipated gives expression to the energy contained within each experience of loss and reclaims something precious in the process. Reflections on acknowledging what you hold include:

Where is there unacknowledged pain in your life?
What is needed to allow the movement and release of
    your pain?
What will you recover by setting down these emotional
    burdens?

What else is held in your womb space that desires acknowledgment?

### Difficult Birth Experiences and Other Events Related to the Female Body

When a woman gives birth in the manner she desires, feeling fully supported while doing so, she more joyfully inhabits her body and her motherhood. The same is true of her first menstruation and her first sexual experience: if these and other bodily events are positive, they further enhance a woman's relationship with her body and her experience of being a woman. If these experiences are negative or traumatic, they can become sources of shame or places she learns to avoid, blocking her root vitality. I have sat with women, massaging the muscles of the pelvic bowl while they remembered a difficult birth or other painful root experience. I encourage them to look for where the energy of the root became blocked in some way and to utilize the womb and ovaries to restore the creative flow in their core. By working in the root and going deep within the energy of the pelvic bowl, they can change the impact of these events on their core—even retrieving vital energy or changing their held energy response to the experience itself—and reconnect to the abundance of their creative center.

### Rediscover Your Womb

When you have released the grief and other pent-up emotions from your pelvic bowl and freed your womb's creative potential, you will delight in this feminine place, which now has the capacity to gestate and support your creations.

### Exercise: Meditation for the Pelvic Bowl

1. Bring awareness down to your pelvic bowl, placing a hand over your low belly.

2. Notice your womb, the center of your pelvic bowl. This is your own space for meeting with spirit. What do you see or feel here? What feels challenging? What brings hope?

3. Sense the connection between this center of your bowl and the space around you. Notice any sensations, images, or thoughts that arise as you sit in your center. How is the energy in your pelvic bowl presently influencing your state of being?

4. Think about what you would you like to hold in your bowl. How will you use your creative potential? What will you offer to your lineage?

5. Breathe deeply into your pelvic bowl. Inhale and fill your entire pelvis with your breath. Exhale and release any tension or places of holding.

6. Inhale, letting the invitations from spirit fill your pelvic bowl. Exhale and release, letting go of anything else. Inhale, bringing spirit into each part of your pelvic bowl. Exhale, trusting your body, surrendering to each movement with spirit.

7. As you bring your visualization to a close, remember that the pelvic bowl is where you draw energy for your creative life. Offer gratitude to your womb, the mother place of your creations.

We take better care of what we claim for ourselves. Spend time in your womb and see what is held in your mother place. Set down the burdens you have carried for so long you have forgotten why they are there. Find the regions that are difficult for you to recognize as your own and open yourself there to spirit. Wherever you have buried your creative impulses under the weight of ancient grief or learned to nurture only the expectations of others, you have feminine ground to reclaim.

## Recognize Patterns of Power Loss

To fully own the creative potential of your uterus, you must know how to access the range of your uterine or feminine power. Because most women are disconnected from the womb space, patterns of power loss are the norm, but the energetic imbalances in the uterus will teach you how you are losing your feminine power. When you restore balance in the uterus, you will also remember the power of your root place.

### Excess Held Energy: Resisting a Creative Movement

One form of uterine energetic imbalance is excess holding. With the pattern of excess uterine holding, a woman overworks her uterus's ability to contain energy. She has difficulty making transitions and trusting the natural creative flow. Like a painter who has to keep fiddling with her painting, a woman keeps gestating her creations rather than finishing one creative cycle and then moving on to the next. The uterus maintains a holding pattern rather than naturally moving between the periods of gathering and release that are part of each creative cycle.

Holding excess uterine energy inhibits a woman's ability to release her creations. It may prevent the release of the placenta and the energy of birth. A woman holds onto her creations and resists the release that is part of each creative movement. She may hold on to a creation because she fears the change or loss, when actually she will receive her bounty in unexpected ways when her creation is given life and shared with a community. She may believe that her creative energy is limited, unaware of its potential for restoration with every completed creative cycle. Because the source of her creative energy is a place of scarcity, her uterine power is held back instead of supporting her and her creations.

When a woman restrains her creative essence, she ultimately limits the expansive nature of her releasing energy. During child-birth, a woman must surrender to the opening of her womb in order to birth her baby. The more she is able to trust her womb, the less resistance she will encounter. When a woman's uterus is fully open, or dilated, birth energy pours through her root. In the same manner, if a woman can allow the opening and release of energy from her womb even while feeling afraid or challenged by a creative experience, she allows the energy to move through her body and expand her potential. In this way, rather than restraining her creative essence, she meets each moment with her full presence.

Excess uterine holding causes stagnation in the pelvic space. When a woman is unable to clear the energy of her uterus on a reg-ular basis, she accumulates stagnant energy in her core, and that buildup creates physical tension in the pelvic bowl. As a result of pelvic tension and uterine holding, a woman may also have dark menstrual blood, prolonged cycles, stagnant creativity, and increased premenstrual symptoms. Even after menopause, these tension pat-terns may cause her to experience difficulty with digestion, constipation, pelvic or abdominal pain, and diminished vitality. In her life, she may tend to hold onto relationships that are not fulfill-ing, sabotage opportunities for growth, or even avoid cleaning out closets, resisting the natural movement of transition.

To make your life or energy more full and to support your body in having healthy menstrual and transition cycles, look for the patterns of greatest holding and restriction in your female body or other feminine realms. Your feminine vitality is limited by the ways you hold yourself back. Expand beyond these limitations— these places of holding—and discover your true potential. Notice the unexpected ways in which you restore your uterine power and gain access to the resources of your whole wild feminine landscape.

## Women's Stories: Making a Full Transition

Ann came for postpartum healing two months after her second child was born. As I worked on her body, she told the story of her child's birth—her pelvic muscles contracting and her breathing quickening as she described the pushing phase of labor. Since this was her second child, she had expected him to be born quickly. Ann was surprised and frustrated by her difficulty at the end of labor.

Touching Ann's pelvic floor muscles, I found an increased level of tension throughout her vagina and nearby musculature. As I massaged away the tension in her root, she was reminded of the place her baby's body had recently passed. Focusing on her pelvis in this way, Ann recalled the overwhelming thoughts and emotions at the end of her son's birth. She had been exhausted and worried, wondering how she would be able to mother two children, meet both of their needs, and still take care of herself as well.

She felt that this doubt about her mothering capacity had slowed the progress of her labor. However, at the time of her son's birth, she could not articulate her concerns, nor did she know how to address them. Ann delivered her son by sheer will rather than a conscious letting go. After her son was born, she forgot the intensity of her feelings in the process of caring for her new baby and toddler.

Now, with her attention returned to the pelvic space, she remembered her previous sense of being overwhelmed. I explained to Ann that her uterus was still in a pattern of holding, rather than the mode of releasing that typically occurs after childbirth. It was as if her body was trying to cope with an increase in mothering demands by holding everything together. I had seen this same pattern of excess uterine holding in several women who were overwhelmed by their work, regardless of profession.

When a woman's external demands change or increase, she often holds tension in the pelvic space as a result. However, this core tension actually reduces her ability to take care of extra children or projects. Continuous holding of uterine energy brings her pelvic energy to maximum capacity; any extra mothering loads will easily overwhelm her energy system. However, when she uses the ability of her uterus to release excess energy, a woman will find that her body is relaxed at the core. As a result, she feels significantly more balanced and capable in all her creative endeavors.

Because she continued to hold uterine energy after the birth of her baby, Ann was unable to receive the influx of energy that accompanies the birth process, or any creative transition. By holding back at a time of uterine release, she was also resisting the energetic completion of this birth event. Faced with increased demands on her energy, she was unable to access her mothering reserves.

To assist Ann in releasing the energy held in her uterus, I guided her through a breathing and visualization exercise. She imagined a stream of water flowing from her uterus into the earth. I encouraged her to allow herself to be carried by the tide of energy from her child's birth. To receive the sustenance of the powerful life-force energy of birth, Ann had to be willing to let go completely, to surrender her old identity as the mother of one child. With each exhalation of breath, she relaxed the tension in her uterus and pelvic area, allowing the energy from her child's birth to move through her body.

Initially, as Ann's uterus began to release, her pelvic space filled with heat. By trusting the energetic movement of her body, she felt the outpouring of uterine energy that naturally accompanies childbirth. After several minutes of clearing excess energy and uterine holding, the heat dissipated and her pelvic tension decreased to a healthy baseline tone. By allowing her uterus a full release, Ann enabled her womb to restore itself after the intensity of sustaining a prolonged gestation. Because Ann was no longer resisting the natural energy flow in her body, her creative energy was also now available to provide support for herself and her mothering.

At the end of our session, Ann felt calm and peaceful. Accustomed to being a high achiever, she realized that she needed to adjust her expectations of herself as the nurturer of two children. She also recognized that not attempting to meet every one of her family's demands and acknowledging the capacity of her partner would provide an opportunity for growth and change in their dynamics as a whole. Even though Ann recognized the benefits of these changes, she also noticed a sense of grief in accepting this transition.

During the next several weeks, she spent a few minutes each day breathing from her womb, releasing the energetic tension in her pelvic bowl. Connecting with her body helped her recognize the grief and other feelings that were part of her transition process. Rather than avoiding her grief or overwhelming feelings, she learned to recognize them as a signal for her to take care of herself and attend to her womb space. By intentionally releasing energy from her core, Ann restored an energetic balance in her body. She felt more capable and centered, able to experience the joy of her changing family and to step into her potential for embracing the change in her life.

## Excess Releasing Energy: Relinquishing the Creative Desire

Another pattern of uterine energetic imbalance is excess releasing. When a woman excessively releases energy, she frequently abandons her personal projects or relinquishes her creative impulses. She gives up her creative dreams, hesitant to be seen as either a success or a failure. She may appear creatively ambitious and be involved in many arenas. But external pressures, rather than her own inner desires, create her goals. As a result, she has no sense of ownership regarding her creative potential.

Lacking clear direction for her creative energy, a woman with this pattern frequently involves herself in work she is not truly invested in. With a continual outpouring of unfocused energy, her uterus depletes itself. Physical symptoms of excess uterine releasing include prolonged bleeding with menstruation, a sense of fatigue, and difficulty engaging the pelvic muscles. When a woman's creative essence is not aligned with her creations, she repeatedly drains her energy and disappoints her own feminine self.

To acknowledge a pattern of excessively releasing uterine energy, reexamine dreams or aspirations you have unintentionally let go. Think of times you have given away your creative potential and refocus the energy of your mother place. Learn to recognize the impulses of your own creative essence. The energy of your womb is meant to support you and your own creations.

### Exercise: Directing Your Creative Energy

1. Reflection: Reflect on the past seven years of your life in relation to your creative energy. On a piece of paper, list one major creation or creative event for each year. Notice how each year felt in terms of creative blocks or creative flow. Reflect on your relationship to your body during these same times.

2. Ritual: On the same piece of paper, write three creative dreams that you want to work on in the coming year. Choose one of these creative dreams to focus on, the one that brings a sense of core delight. On another piece of paper, draw an image or use free-flowing words to describe this particular creative dream. When you are finished, hold this paper con-

taining the seed of your creative vision in your hands while closing your eyes and focusing on your womb. Ask your womb what physical, energetic, and spiritual support will assist this seed to take root in your life. Write down any helpful information and keep it as a tangible reminder of how to direct your creative energy in alignment with your core.

### Women's Stories: Reclaiming Her Vibrancy

Jane came to address some pelvic concerns arising with menopause and sought to reconnect with her vibrancy. She had found her niche in a corporate career, which provided both creative challenge and an outlet for her dynamic nature. But as she prepared herself for retirement and felt the menopausal changes within her body, she grew more disconnected from her own vitality.

In her pelvic muscle assessment, Jane had more tone on the right side, which is often typical for someone oriented to the outer working world, but this tone had an underlying tension pattern that was restricting her core blood and energy flow. She also had a lack of tone on the left side, meaning she had room to cultivate this part of her pelvis and core energy field. Her vaginal canal was dry. Jane had noticed an increase in vaginal dryness that caused a sensitivity with intercourse and even daily discomfort, but she had assumed it was an expected outcome from the hormonal changes of menopause. However, pelvic imbalances will always intensify the effects of hormonal shifts.

I began vaginal massage to stimulate core cellular regeneration and encouraged Jane to breathe toward her center. She was used to focusing only externally, so it felt quite foreign for her to turn her attention inward. I invited her to sense the strong vital flow of her creative energy that had nurtured her successful career. By turning this powerful energy toward her center, she could recharge her own vitality.

Noticing her core, Jane recognized a truth for herself. She had been disassociating from her body in an attempt to avoid the negative stereotypes that portray a woman as less radiant with age. But this subtle disconnection from herself had actually contributed to a sense of herself as diminishing; she had lost touch with her own creative center. By returning to her body, she would reaffirm her dynamic nature regardless of her stage in life. Negative stereotypes and ideas about the female body are what restrict a woman's radiance. When a woman feels her body, and her creative energy, she knows the truth of her beauty.

With the internal massage, Jane could feel the warmth and suppleness return to her pelvic muscles. She noted how it was just like having a facial, with massage on the hardworking but often forgotten parts of the body. Our bodies always benefit from thoughtful care, and the pelvic bowl is no different. With a little vaginal self-massage, Jane found that her pelvic muscles felt more supple and her vagina was more lubricated on a regular basis. Massage was helping her to increase the core blood and energy flow that enhances cellular and hormonal circulation. With a renewed inner focus, Jane recovered the vibrancy that would sustain and inspire her next phase of life.

## Restore Your Feminine Power

By identifying and addressing the imbalances in your uterine energy, you restore the feminine power of your womb. For example, if you feel a scarcity in your life (lack of emotional support, no time to rest, financial strain) your uterine holding energy will often increase to a point of imbalance. Although this is a natural response to fear and insecurity, the tension in your core prevents you from claiming the abundance of your creative feminine power. The antidote to uterine holding is surrendering control and accepting the support you receive, from both the energy within and external sources in your life. Even when this process results in unexpected outcomes, it leads you to the next phase of your growth.

To change your uterine energy from a pattern of holding to one of letting go, create a mantra. The rhythmic and repetitive words of a mantra, like prayer, serve as an energetic bridge; they provide support for creating new energetic and physical patterns. For example, repeating *I release my fear of being alone to embrace the love around me*, may help the root of the body to soften and the uterus to release its tension and energy. Saying a mantra with a specific intention invites your energy to change form.

Notice your tendency to hold or release uterine energy, and allow yourself to experiment with new ways of being in your core. The following exercise may assist you to discover your uterine energy patterns.

### Exercise: Uterine Energy Patterns

1. Reflection: Divide a piece of paper in half. On one side, draw a symbol of your uterus with an arrow pointing in to represent times of holding or gestation. List everything you can think of that you have nurtured or held. On the other side, draw the same symbol for your uterus with an arrow pointing out to represent times of release; list everything you have cleared or given birth to. Look at the two lists and notice the patterns of holding or letting go in your life. Think about times you have been able to access your feminine power or times you have been stuck in a pattern of imbalance. Contemplate how to restore your uterine balance and feminine power.

2. Ritual: Find or create a small bowl to represent your uterus and place it on an altar or designated place. Surround it with

written words or objects that reflect and inspire your creative
essence, and fill it with intentions for your present creative
desires; tend to or evolve these over time. Consciously claim
and cultivate the energy of your womb space, the heart of
your feminine power.

Restoring uterine balance requires that you regularly access
both the holding and releasing energies of your uterus. If you
notice a tendency toward either holding or releasing, practice the
opposing energy movement. Release an emotional situation you
were previously holding on to or reclaim a project you were about
to let go.

Look for habits that sustain energetic imbalances and begin to
change them. You may have excess uterine holding in response to
an unmet need or a sense of compromised safety. Excess releasing
energy may arise when you are playing down your success (so that
others are not threatened by your abilities) or denying your own
needs. Whatever the cause of these imbalances, notice when they
occur—and reclaim your feminine power.

## Hone the Power in Your Womb

In the days after my miscarriage, I knew I would have another child
born at that time the next year. I felt this knowing in my body, a
certainty I had rarely experienced, and I followed the promptings
of my womb, waiting to open the spirit door again until it felt right.
With my body as a guide, my husband and I began to consciously
conceive our second child.

A positive pregnancy test several weeks later confirmed my
baby's pending arrival, but my older son had already alerted me to
the potential in my womb. Not yet three years old, my son looked
at my belly and said, "Mama, a baby is coming. He is my brother.
I have not seen him in a long time; I will be so glad to see him." His

brother was born in early August the following year, three days before the anniversary of my miscarriage.

In my desire to contact the baby I lost, I gave my womb constant attention in the weeks following my miscarriage. Having worked on the root of my body with vaginal massage and the energy of my organs through breath, visualization, and ritual, I was deeply connected to my female body. I believe this connection to my pelvic bowl, even in the midst of my grief, enabled me to know (and perhaps my older son to sense) that another child was coming. This root connection also allowed me to bond immediately, without hesitation, even in the earliest days of conception. I fully trusted my womb and the path of this next creation. The womb is powerful because it is sacred space, a place to commune with spirit and receive the intuitive wisdom and support that arises from such direct encounters with the spiritual realm.

## The Energy of Menstruation

One way to honor the female body as sacred is to match the pace of your life to the rhythmic cycle of the womb. In its most natural state, the menstrual cycle is twenty-eight days long, just like the moon cycle: the uterus is either building or shedding its blood in relationship to the moon's waxing and waning. The menstrual cycle often correlates with the moon because hormonal regulation of fertility is affected by exposure to light. Particularly in the absence of the artificial light of cities, the female body responds to the changes in light that occur with the different phases of the moon. A woman may look to the changes of the moon or the signals from her body to recognize patterns in her creative cycle.

With menopause, a woman is said to contain all her energy and wisdom internally as she moves into her time as an elder. The women in my practice who are transitioning into menopause often begin to reevaluate what they want for themselves. No longer pouring energy into the caretaking of others, they have more energy for their personal lives. By learning to read the creative energy within the body, they can still notice an inner movement that correlates to their own creative cycle, a call from the body to clear or gather energy in the womb space.

Additionally, the energy of menstruation is a physical reflection of the uterine capacity to hold or release. Remembering to access this potential for holding and releasing energy in the body, even when a woman is no longer having a physical cycle, is beneficial for any life transition she makes. Changing jobs, reinventing or dissolving a marriage, creating a new partnership, sending a child off to college, completing a major project, losing a parent, facing a serious illness, making a new home: all major life events require that we choose what to hold or release in order to make a complete transition.

The changes in the female body and menstrual cycle also correlate to changes in a woman's energetic capacity. When building a menstrual lining, a woman may feel bold and prepared for new challenges. Her energy is robust and full, and she has more energetic support from her body. When bleeding or shedding this lining, she may want to retreat from the demands of the outer world. When releasing menstrual blood, a woman's energetic core is more open, so she can release core energy and receive intuitive guidance, and this sensitizes her being. Too much busyness or outer focus during the initial part of menstruation diminishes the body's inherent ability to clear and rebalance core energy. It is wise and respectful to follow the rhythms of the female body and the corresponding impulses for emotional and creative expansion or retreat.

As women begin to use the alternating cycles of uterine energy in everyday life, their menstrual cycles may change. In my practice, women have reported shorter and less painful menstrual cycles as they regain greater pelvic balance. Their menstrual blood becomes a brighter red, and they notice fewer premenstrual symptoms. By consciously accessing the natural flow of their female energy systems, women find that their menstrual cycles are able to clear their pelvic energies more efficiently. They feel productive and restored, more in sync with their own creative pace.

In the full demands of life, bleeding every month can still feel like a burden. With all that I have to accomplish in a given day in tending a women's healthcare practice and three children, I often greet my own bleeding time with a sigh. However, I recognize the importance of bleeding to my energetic and physical health and accept this process as an integral part of my body's cleansing and renewal. In my blood I am shedding a physical and energetic layer in preparation for the next creative cycle. I speak about this process to my children: the importance of bleeding, my need to align my energy to my cycle, and the beautiful blood that served as their initial nourishment. In speaking with honor and respect about the menstrual cycle, I am creating an early imprint of the body as sacred, reprogramming the cultural messages of shame.

Be conscious of your body by selecting natural menstrual products free of bleach, fragrances, plastics, and other chemicals that are toxic to the sensitive vaginal and pelvic tissues and actually interfere with the body's natural cleansing process. Natural sea sponges, menstrual cups, and cloth pads are all more gentle to your body. Allowing menstrual blood to flow for part of the cycle, rather than exclusively using tampons, is also helpful to encourage pelvic energy flow. If you experience pain and significant cramping with your menstrual cycle, it is often a sign that you have layers of tension in the abdomen inhibiting the natural contractions of the uterus or ovaries. Menstruation and ovulation should not be painful. Find a practitioner of Maya Abdominal Massage (the Arvigo Techniques) on the web. Maya massage may reduce tension in the abdomen and realign the uterus, often alleviating menstrual or ovulation pain altogether.

When you are menstruating, making time for self-care and solitary retreat will assist your body in clarifying the energy of your pelvic bowl.

## Exercise: Conscious Menstruation

1. Uterine release: During a time of release in your body, you most easily release words, thoughts, or other ways of using your creative energy that no longer serve your well-being. Honor your sacred blood; your own cells began life in the protective layer of womb blood. When you are bleeding, think about what you are shedding. Give yourself permission to release any worn-out attitudes or energies from your body and mind. Visualizing your womb, you may say, "I release anything that is no longer necessary. I release completely, trusting that I have what I need." Make some quiet space for your release, focusing on the base of your bowl and feeling a connection to the earth where your bowl can release. Receive the intuitive energies that are available to you in this more open time.

2. Uterine holding: When your uterus is in a state of holding, notice the change in your pelvic bowl. The energy building in your core is a source of strength, ready to gestate whatever enlivens you as a woman. Visualizing your womb, you may say, "I embrace my creative dreams. I embrace my full creative essence." Awaken to your body's rhythms; access the potential they contain for you.

### Women's Stories: Finding a Place to Rest

When Diane came to see me, she was looking for direction in her life. She felt aimless and was unsure of how to access or direct her creative essence. If a woman needs specific answers for herself, I encourage her to connect with her womb, the core of her feminine wisdom. Guiding Diane to her pelvic space, and her uterine energy, I discovered part of her difficulty. Balanced uterine energy should either be full and steady, indicating a time of gestation, or it should flow like a river, indicating a time of release. Diane's uterine energy was erratic and unsteady.

Although it was hard for her to stay focused on her uterus in the midst of its chaotic energy pattern, it was exactly what she needed to do. Bringing a woman into a busy energy pattern reminds me of teaching my sons to step onto an escalator. The rushing energy is intimidating at first. It requires a moment of faith to leap into the moving energy and be carried by it. Diane's uterus felt as if it was racing, and she recognized that her core energy was a reflection of her hectic daily life. She tended to work continuously, without regard for her true desires or the natural energy flow in her body. At first Diane felt overwhelmed by the intensity of this frenetic energy, but by staying focused on the discomfort in her center, she gradually gained a foothold and was able to sit in her womb space.

When Diane initially encountered the frantic pace of her womb energy, her instinct was to ignore this sense of agitation in herself. But by paying attention to the agitation, she felt a release and her pelvic energy began to slow. Although women often avoid energy blocks and burdens in the core, it is precisely by attending to these uncomfortable sensations, with quiet awareness, that the energy pattern begins to change and the energy block clears. After the release in her body, Diane experienced a sense of inner calm with a slower pace in her center. Gradually, a natural womb rhythm began. She noticed that she felt stronger, drawing from a more sustainable energy pattern. Diane could now access the flow of her uterine energy to guide her creative movements and provide her creative direction.

## Understanding the Creative Nature of the Female Body

As the center of the pelvic bowl, the energy of the uterus reminds us of our innate creative potential as women. We can use it to align our own creative energies and to understand the nuances of the greater patterns of creative flow in our lives. When something appears as creative stagnation, focusing on the center can assist us in determining whether there is an imbalance in our energy, an area in need of healing, or a more global pattern of flow where the greater energies are building and aligning as part of a cycle in a broader process. There are cycles of growth and transition for us as individuals, and in the collective. Attuning to the center increases our alignment with our own inner cycles and focuses our creative energy to be in sync with the creative whole as well.

Another challenge for us as a community is that we are continuously exposed to environmental toxins, and our bodies are attempting to clear these exposures. Both physically—with an abundance of lymph nodes and vaginal and uterine fluids—but also energetically, the pelvic bowl plays an essential role in this clearing. We can assist our bodies by taking care of the pelvic bowl, reducing physical and energetic stagnation with holistic and integrative pelvic self-care. Likewise, we can use the capacity of the bowl when we undergo any type of medical procedure. With the increasing identification of uterine and ovarian cysts that reveal cellular changes or other challenges for the body, women may need to combine Western medicine techniques such as surgery with more holistic bodywork and energy medicine tools. For example, I had a facial surgery to remove a skin cancer, and I elected to have the surgery, but I also worked with my pelvic energy to clear my energetic field and call in supportive energies during the procedure to assist the healing process. Increasing our daily presence in the pelvic bowl, we can align with the sacred in our most challenging times of healing or to savor a lighthearted moment. Accessing our creative potential in response to our daily lives is how we take our conceptual knowledge and actually embody our sacredness.

Increasing presence in the pelvic bowl strengthens our connection and energy flow with the earth. We used to bleed and even give birth (or be born) directly onto the earth. Remembering this connection, we are better able to receive nourishment from this energetic grounding. This provides a strong center for our bodies to align with and gives support to our relationships. In my home life, I have noted that my German shepherd listens more readily, my parrot is calmer, and my children more centered themselves when I am fully present and balanced in my bowl. Again, women often look outside of themselves for the perfect partner, ideal weight, or right job in hopes of establishing a sense of ease without realizing that aligning with the center is a key step in finding what they seek.

## Gather Your Uterine Energy

Your uterine ability to gather and hold energy is a profound resource. You may choose how and when to utilize your gestational capacity, and being conscious in this process is a way of honoring yourself as a woman and cultivating your own creative dreams. If you gather its energy when your female body is in a natural state of holding, it will support you in any creative endeavor. Your internal sense of energetic vitality—often correlating with ovulation, the full moon, or your own inner sense—indicates that your root is preparing to hold and gestate energy.

Attune yourself to the natural rhythm of your uterus by noticing when you feel resilient and capable. Prepare to start a new project, activate a conscious change for yourself, or make a bold move. Remember to hold what is good, expanding your potential to sustain a joy-filled life. Use the following exercise to gather your uterine energy.

### Exercise: Gathering Uterine Energy

Read the exercise through first, and then close your eyes to begin. Find a comfortable position sitting or lying down.

1. Guide your attention internally to your pelvic bowl and notice any sensations that arise. Bring your focus to your uterus at the center of your pelvis. Envision the energy of your uterus extending out in all directions like a full skirt. In a time of natural uterine gathering, your energy feels strong and vibrant. Ask your body what you are gathering energy for and reflect on a word or image that symbolizes this creation.

2. In your mind's eye, walk to the edges of the energetic skirt around your pelvis. See yourself sweeping this energy toward your center, toward your uterus. Walk in a full circle, sweeping your arms around each part of your pelvis.

3. As you gather the energy of your pelvis in toward your center, notice any areas that have been leaking this vital creative energy. Leaks will feel like holes or edges that are difficult to define. These leaks symbolize areas in your life where you are giving away your creative potential, perhaps out of habit or unintentionally. When you pay attention to these holes in the energy field of your bowl, you will discover how you are draining your creative energy. Bring your awareness to these vulnerable regions in order to change patterns that would otherwise deplete your female energy system.

4. Now return to the center of your pelvic space. Notice the circle of energy that surrounds you; this is the uterine energy you are holding. Visualize a specific intention or creation, and then surround it with your creative energy. Focus on these words, images, or colors in your bowl, breathing into your center five to seven times.

5. Offer thanks to your uterus for its sustenance and bring your visualization to a close. Feel the greater energetic support

available for your womb space, creations, and radiant feminine self when you focus on your center.

## Clear the Womb Space

The days when you feel vulnerable, almost transparent, correspond with the release of uterine energy. A period for reflection and restorative retreat, uterine release may correlate with your bleeding time, the new moon, or your inner creative cycle. It is your own internal sense of lower energy that signals an energetic release from your female body. Feeling overloaded or too full also signals the need for uterine release.

The releasing ability of your uterus is a powerful force. When your female body is in a natural state of release, use this power to clarify your womb space. This is the time to change emotional or other self-limiting patterns, release pelvic tension, prepare for a transition, and clear excess energy from your core. Let go of resentments and old patterns of body, mind, and spirit. True forgiveness requires letting go of held energy. You do not need to know what is being released, just give your body permission.

If you are not menstruating, due to lactation or menopause, it is especially important to perform a monthly uterine releasing exercise to prevent energetic imbalances resulting from the lack of a regular period of release. Additionally, releasing your uterine energy before conceiving a child will clear your pelvic space and prepare you to receive an incoming soul. But during pregnancy, you do not need a regular uterine releasing exercise because you are in a time of sustained uterine holding. Release your uterine energy to restore balance in your core after a birth process, including the birth of a miscarriage. In my own experience, working with the releasing capacity of my uterus allowed me to complete a miscarriage at home with the natural contractions of my body.

Releasing uterine energy can also assist major life changes or act as a form of self-care to clear accumulated energy. Go and sit directly on the earth to support your womb in clearing the energetic charge that the body accumulates from electronics and the hectic pace of life. When you begin to clear the energy of your womb space, you may realize that many others are asking to be sustained by your creative energy. Your own self, your creations, your children, and only those whom you choose are meant to be nourished by the energy of your bowl. Clear your bowl of all other excess energy and unintentional caretaking duties, and you will also be clearer about how you desire to direct your creative energy. Pay attention to the signals from your body during a time of uterine release to gain access to the intuitive insight that accompanies the rhythmic movements of the womb.

### Exercise: Clearing the Womb Space

Read the exercise through first. Find a comfortable position sitting or lying down, and then close your eyes to begin.

1. Guide your attention to your pelvic bowl and the energy of your core. Notice any sensations that arise. Then bring your focus to your uterus at the center of your pelvis. Notice what you are preparing to release, whether you are completing the gestation of a creative project or intentionally clearing a specific energy.

2. Take in a full breath, and then exhale. As you release your breath, invite your womb to begin its release. Visualize the energy—as a stream of water, light, or your menstrual blood—leaving your womb and going down into the earth. Look for any hesitation or resistance to this clearing, and release each area of resistance with your breath. Trust your body's release, knowing that you will still have the creative energy you need.

3. Acknowledge any creations that are being released. Find a place in your heart or life for those that will continue to nourish you, and set down those that are done—letting this energy flow. Visualize the energy leaving your uterus and moving out into the world with each exhalation of your breath. Continue for as long as needed for a full release.

4. Now continue to release excess energy or any energy that does not presently serve you. Visualize this energy leaving your body and going down into the fiery core of the earth. With each exhalation, feel your uterus letting go. Set your intention for this release. How can you receive the blessing of what is leaving or changing at this time? What is your womb revealing about your feminine self? Continue as long as needed for a full release (some energy may continue to trickle, but you will feel lighter in your core).

5. Notice any areas of tension in your body, including your face, torso, pelvic bowl, arms, or legs; release from each area. Repeat five to seven times or until your entire body's release feels complete. Then allow the energy of the earth to move up through your legs and into your bowl to revitalize and renew your creative core.

6. Offer gratitude to your womb for its assistance and connection to the earth, and bring your visualization to a close. Notice any changes in your womb space, your sense of clarity, and your overall feeling of fullness.

## Listen to Your Womb

The womb has a wealth of wisdom for you as a woman. Listen to her guidance on how to nourish yourself, build your creations, connect with spirit, and follow your creative rhythms. Listen to your womb whether or not you have birthed babies or have moved into menopause. Even if you have had a hysterectomy, the powerful energy center of your womb is still contained within the core of your pelvic bowl. This is the mother, your connection to the earth and the energy for all that you will create in this life. Listen to your womb in regard to partners, birth control, menstrual products, and all other creative decisions. It is the wisest place in your center.

## Live from Your Creative Center

Your womb is a place of connection with spirit and creativity, and its internal rhythm and energy provides essential guidance for living a creative life. Just as there are monthly changes in uterine energy, you may also notice daily and even yearly cycles of creative energy that alternate between expansive movement and restorative stillness. These cycles are the basis of your own cycle of fertility. Moving in sync with the creative rhythms of your body, you hone the creative power in your womb.

To be creative in a sustainable manner, learn to cultivate your creativity like a farmer cultivates her crop: each harvest represents many days, and even seasons, of working with the land. My ability to write and sustain a women's health practice, in the midst of birthing and nurturing my children, was possible because I approached my creative life in a cyclical manner. I tended to my creations by following my own monthly and annual creative cycles. I alternated between writing and working, caring for my children, and taking care of myself in an organic, fluid way. I continue to engage my creative energy from an inner rhythm, sometimes holding a particular piece of healing or a creation with focused intention, and then letting go of my focus and restoring order to my greater environment. Always moving from my core or returning to my center when feeling out of balance, I follow the flow of my inner rhythms through periods of quiet, internal retreat, and active times of harvest.

Western culture tends to disregard natural rhythms of the creative process, requiring continuous output regardless of season. However, when you attune to your own cycle of fertility, you can access the energetic support corresponding to the rhythms of your female body. Following your own inner rhythms through a full creative cycle will enhance both your capacity to create and the sustenance you receive from the creative process.

### Exercise: Embracing a Full Creative Cycle

Choose one of your creative dreams or inspirations and ponder how to support its growth by envisioning a full creative cycle. Some cycles may be completed in a few weeks while others may take several years, depending on the creation. Rather than setting a required period of time to achieve a full creative cycle, there should be a natural flow that results in a tangible harvest and a sense of completion.

1. Groundwork: Reflect on the creative dream you have chosen for this exercise. What type of preparation do you need to begin planting the seeds of your creative dream? What needs to be cleared in order to make room for your creation?

2. Nourishment: Think about the nourishment that will encourage the growth of these seeds. Do you need to take a class and learn new skills, engage in an activity that inspires you, or nurture your own creative center in some way?

3. Cultivation: Imagine the resources available in your community and how they might assist you to tend this creative crop. How might you network or gather with others to be inspired or do the work of cultivating your creations?

4. Harvest: Consider a tangible place that will mark a full creative cycle. Celebrating your creative harvest allows you to be nourished by the fruits of your labor. How will you celebrate and share your bounty with others?

5. Fallow Time: The downtime that follows a creative burst is essential for replenishing your creative energy and gaining insight for planting your next creative seeds. Do you take regular time for solitude and rest?

As you rediscover your natural womb and creative cycles, you give support to your whole female body. Tend your home and hearth with care; honor your inner sanctuaries. Make vibrant and visible creations that express your unique essence. With her maternal nature, the uterus asks that we take care of ourselves and give life to our heartfelt creations. Follow her lead from restorative retreat to expansive creation, and you will prepare a womb—and a life—that is ready for your own planting.

*May you find the purpose of your creative rhythms.*

SIX

# Transforming
# Your Inheritance

*For each of us, our body represents a point in time on a long flow*
*of life energy that includes the past energy of our ancestors and the*
*energy of those who will come after us. This chapter explains how*
*to tap into this flow even where there is family pain or unknown*
*lineage. Working with lineage patterns, we heal ourselves and restore*
*the full flow of our rightful energy to do our creative work.*
*Each of us doing this work also heals and restores the*
*energy flow of the community. Finding our ability*
*to create within a collective context is what*
*ultimately returns the purpose to our lives.*

)am sitting by the river. In the foothills of the Appalachians, I have
come to find my father line. I have a bodily sense of my maternal
lineage, a familiar stir of their restless bones in myself, but I never
knew my father's family. I lived far from the land where they made
their home, and I can detect no imprint of their lives within my own.

My second son and I have embarked on a day trip from New
York City to roam a rural county in eastern Pennsylvania. Several
years have passed since my wild feminine flight across the country to
visit my New York City girlfriend. Time has made its passage known.
My friend has become a mother; she has a daughter of her own. The
baby whose milk filled my breasts during that journey now stands
beside me, throwing one black rock after another into the water.

Tired of driving, we have parked our car next to a railroad tres-tle and followed a trail that led to a river. My son delights in this river, perfectly sized for skipping stones and for other boyhood adventures. I imagine my paternal grandfather as a boy, fishing for his dinner. His mother, my great-grandmother, died when he was six, during a flu epidemic that swept through the mountain valley one hard winter. An unborn baby died with her. My grandfather would have been the same age as my oldest son, too young to be so unsheltered in the world.

I have a paper with the names and birth dates of all ten of my great-grandmother's children. My grandfather's name is there, her seventh child. Some of the children's deaths are recorded: two at birth and two a few short years after being born. I have one faded picture of my great-grandmother, and I look at her sepia face and think of her body, birthing and caring for her many children, while she had to bury some of them too. It gives me reason to pause. I offer a moment of silence for the weariness that must have even-tually taken her from this life.

My son and I spend the day exploring the region where my rel-atives, most of whom have died, once lived. I had no clear direction but want to see and touch the land where they lived for generations. What surprises me most of all is how familiar it seems. Though I have never been here before, I know this landscape. I pass porches with roughly hewn benches just like the ones I have collected in my Oregon home. The large wooden bowl in my kitchen and my fondness for hand-carved tools and weathered barns belong to the scenery of this place.

I came here to find what was lost, only to discover that it was with me all along. I carry my father's line, but not until traveling my ancestral ground could I recognize its lineage as my own.

On the drive back to the city, my son sleeps as the countryside disappears behind us. Later I will call my father and share our jour-ney into the county of his father's family. He tells me that I was near the small town where my grandfather was born. When I find this town on the map, I am surprised to see the same river where we ended our journey.

Tracing the curve of its line, I see how the river winds from where my son and I stood, flowing two miles downstream, to the place of my grandfather's birth. Rather than planning the details of our day, I had followed the natural rhythm that led us to the banks of this small river. It could have been any river, but it was the one my grandfather would have known. It was there that I felt his presence most vividly. In a land where I had never been, I somehow found my way. I reach for the smooth stone in my pocket, the one I lifted from the riverbank, and hold a piece of my grandfather's river. This same river flows through me.

## Defining Lines: The Energy of Lineage

The lines we travel most frequently—words spoken, habits of living, company kept—eventually define the range of our lives. Repetition has power because it builds energy over time. When something is repeated—thoughts, actions, movement patterns, and so on—it takes on a structure (a pattern) that is energetic at its core. This is how rituals and traditions become meaningful: their repetition gives them a tangible form. Lineage is passed on in this same manner. The ways we use our creative potential, the languages we speak, the crops we grow, the meals we make, the traditions we celebrate all gather energy, especially when passed parent to child over several generations.

Disruptions in our bodily energy flow often result from broken family lines that were not fully repaired or are in need of new structures. When our ancestors immigrated, or were displaced, they had to make new lives for themselves, often losing ties with the culture and places of their homelands. The stress of moving to a new land is like the effort of breaking ground for the first time; it takes many seasons and a cooperative fate to produce an abundant crop. If the land differs greatly from the one left behind, it can take several generations to understand how to work with the soil, the climate, and the people to build community and other forms of sustenance again. There is loss in such transitions, and loss of family, tradition, and the sense of belonging to a place and a people must be grieved by someone.

A woman may look to the energy of her lineage to understand where to continue the work of her ancestors. The energy of her father and mother lines stretch out behind her body. The energy of her father's family stands behind her on the right side. The energy of her mother's family stands behind her on the left side. The potential of each lineage is hers to own if she will recognize and work with her inheritance.

## Our Bodies Carry Lineage
Delving into the root, we discover the body memory, a deep current that awaits our attention. Formed in the womb, our bodies imprint the legacy of our lineage, the grief and hope of each generation. In reconnecting to the internal rhythm of the female body, we encounter the lineage patterns we carry regarding our creativity as women.

In the past fifty years, women have achieved opportunities for professional success, yet we still embody patterns from our lineage that define and limit our feminine range. A woman's understanding of her femininity is shaped by the lives of those who came before her. While we typically look outside of ourselves to change this inheritance, a woman is best able to choose how she cultivates her creative essence when she examines and redefines her internal and bodily relationship to the feminine.

If womanhood is perceived as a hardship, there are many ways a woman may seek to change her own fate. As we have seen in previous stories, for example, the daughter of a self-sacrificing mother might pursue a career and avoid having children, intent on escaping the burdens encountered in the home. However, this woman still engaged her creative nature in a manner that echoed her mother's approach to life. The act of living in the female form is passed from mother to daughter. The daughter may continue the inherited energetic pattern of her lineage by sacrificing herself in some way, just as her mother did. Altering external circumstances will not help a woman when unsustainable energy patterns remain in her body.

Working with women in my practice, I have seen how the pelvic bowl contains a record of a woman's relationship to the feminine. The lineage she carries, the ways that women and men of her line responded to the feminine in their own lives, is reflected in the energy patterns of her pelvic bowl. The vitality of her uterine and ovarian energies, the emotional energy patterns, and the balance of masculine and feminine in her core, will reflect the ways creative energy was accessed or blocked in her family line.

By studying the nuances of her creative energy, a woman can begin to nourish herself where she was—or those who came before her were—left unfulfilled or defeated. Some of her ancestors may have struggled with real limitations like poverty, war, grave illness, slavery, or traumas that left fractures in her lineage. Even though a woman may not have personally experienced these same events, she may live with a smaller range until she addresses the inherited patterns that convey a sense of danger or scarcity.

A woman may search her own body like a map, rediscovering the places where she, or her ancestors, lost touch with the abundance of their feminine ground. Ponder the changing roles of women—and the record of these changes in your own body—with the following exercise.

### Exercise: Generational Change and the Body Record

1. Visualize yourself as one of your ancestors living in a tribal community. Imagine yourself cooking by the fire, breastfeeding

a child, or gathering roots or berries. What do you smell? What does the earth look like? What else do you notice? Pay attention to your pelvic bowl. How does it feel? Where are you sitting, and what do you notice about the response in your body?

2. Imagine you are a woman during the feminist movement of the 1970s. Where do you see yourself? Are you tending the home or out in the workplace? Do you work in both of these arenas? Notice the sensations in your body. What is happening in your daily life, and how is this reflected in your body and pelvic bowl?

3. See yourself in the present time. How have you shaped your life as a woman? How do you use your creative energy on a daily basis? What fires do you tend? Are you mothering children? Do you have a profession? How are you balancing the inner home and the outer world? How does your body reflect the ways that you are engaging your creative potential?

4. Bring your visualization to a close, giving thanks for the ancestors and the work of those who came before you. Reflect on your observations about each scenario and how they affected your core energy.

Each generation brings progress. The feminist movement liberated women from the roles that restricted their career choices and personal freedom, but it left much to be done regarding the balance of our work and home lives. Women gained access to the working world and professional development, but the more feminine realms—and the nurturing and caregiving roles related to our less visible inner sanctuaries—were often sacrificed in the process. However, when patterns are profoundly dysfunctional, sometimes the only choice is to break them and make repairs later.

The children of the feminist generation, now adults themselves, are reweaving the feminine back into the structures that support our daily routines and the energy we use in our homes, work, gender roles, and how we relate to one another. The next feminist movement is to fully restore our direct connection to the feminine and then re-create a robust and authentic masculine. By exploring emotional patterns, pelvic boundaries, unspoken agreements, and other patterns of energy that have been handed down through our lineage, we discover the ways to receive or transform our inheritance.

## Fear: Find Your Faith

When a woman explores the lines that define her creative range, she will encounter her relationship with fear and faith. If she has trust in the world—a faith in the goodness of others, her connection with spirit, and her own abilities—then her creative range is more expansive than if she is limited by fear. Healthy fear is protective and keeps a woman from harm. But most fear is self-imposed and restricts her capacity to create. For a woman to change her given creative range often requires that she examine her fear and restore a sense of faith in its place. Whether she is bringing a child into the world or embarking on a creative partnership, the line between a woman's fear and her faith draws a boundary, inside which she develops her creations.

Even as I began to write this book, fear shaped my belief of what was possible; I thought I needed the support of a publisher. As a mother of young children and a physical therapist tending a women's health practice, the thought of taking on an extensive writing project without tangible support was daunting. In faith, I sent the initial chapters to an agent in New York who was enthusiastic about the project. Though he sent it to many publishers (in one large batch the day I went into labor with my second son), none of them accepted it.

My faith wavered. I only had faith for this creation in one particular way. I feared that the project would never be completed, and I continued to search for a publisher on my own. But I ran into the same issues my book was designed to address: the split between feminine spirit and female body. The spiritually focused publishers did not publish books about the female body. The feminist presses did not publish spiritual books. The external support that I sought in the publishing industry was unavailable, reflecting a similar divide that I witnessed in the root of the female body.

At the same time, I received support from the women in my midst, my partner, my children, and other workings of spirit. Though I hesitated to trust the path in front of me and had to express my grief for not finding the support I wanted, eventually I stopped trying to find a publisher and concentrated instead on writing. Space opened in unexpected ways as I focused less on fear and more on the creation itself. I chose words and tended them with care; another baby filled my belly and was born. One day, about seven years after I began, a self-published *Wild Feminine* was done. Two years later, I found a publisher for *Wild Feminine* that was forging new ground, bridging the connection between spirit and body. It was work, because a book does not write itself, but the work became the way to spend time in the company of spirit. My faith had grown and with it my capacity for creation; my fear had simply become part of the path.

## The Root Voice of Fear: Wildness Restricted

The root voice of fear is intimidating—it can stop you from living your dreams. It resounds at any hint of change and may strongly insist that you keep silent and remain inside constricting boundaries. The root voice of fear restricts natural energy flow. Sometimes the fear has been in your root so long that you cannot even identify what it might be keeping you from.

Fear builds tension and constriction, rather than allowing for expansion, in the energy pattern and physical structure of the body.

Because the female body is capable of manifesting outwardly what it holds within, constriction in the core may reinforce patterns of emotional, energetic, or financial scarcity based on fear held in the pelvic space. As I have heard women give expression to their root voices, they have voiced fear about connecting to the pelvic bowl, being female, being sensual and sexual, becoming a mother, trusting spirit, taking creative risks, speaking truth, reclaiming their energy, standing their ground, and so on. This fear may be a result of a woman's experience, or it may arise as an accumulation of those fears that have been passed through her lineage. Either way, a woman's fear ultimately reveals where her wild feminine desires its freedom.

Fear is a normal reaction to the difficult situations in our lives, but if held in the body, it interferes with our living. Society has long used fear as a tool to disassociate women from their bodies and their creative potential. Many women who are confident in their own power have been the targets of past or present-day witch hunts. As a result, holding power and embodying full radiance can seem dangerous, causing women to distrust their own bodies. In recovering the power of our bodies and creative energies, we may experience nightmares and intense feelings of fear. However, by meeting each fear with the courage to continue moving and making our own paths, we will fully reclaim our rightful range.

Live your creative dreams and become more radiant, powerful, and expressive by meeting your fear with faith. Notice the subtle ways that you are restricted by fear. Fear arises when opportunities for personal growth present themselves; if you let it stop your progress through life, you continually live with less. When you feel fear, your body may become tense. You may choose to stop, turn around, and never move beyond this fear. Or you may take a breath—inhale faith, exhale fear—and then continue on your way.

Reflections on the root voice of fear include:

Where do you hold fear-based constriction in your body
and life?
Do you see your potential for expansion?
What lineage patterns that you carry are related to fear?
How does your fear reveal your desire for freedom?

*Women's Stories: September 11*

The day after September 11, 2001, I felt the waves of shock that
registered as a layer in the root of our bodies. I had a full schedule of clients to see in my Oregon-based women's health
practice. Normally my focus is to restore balance in the pelvic
bowl, using my physical medicine to massage and align the
internal pelvic muscles. But on this day, I simply tried to make
sense of what I was finding. I helped my clients return to their
center and sort through the signals of chaos ringing in the core.

Working with the first woman, I found that her pelvic
floor muscles were even more tight and painful than when she
initially came to see me. The root energy of her body was
extremely hot, conveying a major stress response. This seemed
coincidental, but appointment after appointment demonstrated
that each woman's pelvic energy and root musculature was
quite altered from the shock of the September 11 tragedy.

With breath, touch, and a radiant sky, the body opens,
partaking fully of the life force. With shock, the breath stops,
the body tenses, the flow of life force is disrupted. Shock, as a
body layer, makes the tissue brittle and rigid—a series of dis-
ordered cells rather than a pulsing and organized form.

We all have shock layers in the root from our individual
pain and tragedy, and I have witnessed many of these layers by
working with women's bodies. A woman's root becomes
physically and energetically activated by personal encounters
that threaten her safety. But the day after September 11 was

the first time I felt a shock pattern that echoed through the body of every client in the same manner: a collective response to a common tragedy.

While these post–September 11 feelings of fear and distress were quite valid, the health and vitality of the vagina and pelvic space are compromised when guarding at such a high level. When a woman's root is in distress, she often avoids connecting with this part of her body without realizing that she is relinquishing her feminine ground, a vital source of energy and nurturance.

I have learned this from working with shock layers in the body: by traveling these layers at a pace that invites breath, the cells begin a movement that will heal the disruption. I have seen that where the trauma layer in the body lies, there also lies an infinite potential for healing. Whenever there is a disruption in the structure of the body or the body of the community, there is also an opening—an invitation to find the breath and follow the movement that arises to honor, to remember, to bear witness, to give life.

## Fear and the Body

The body responds to fear by closing down all but the most vital functions. It goes into a mode of survival, prompting a woman to act out of primitive instinct rather than from her creative capacity. The root of the female body is particularly vulnerable to fear because the base of the pelvic bowl contains the root chakra: the energy center that regulates a woman's core identity and her sense of security. When she feels safe, a woman's pelvic muscles relax and she feels her connection to life, her place of belonging. When she is afraid, the energy of her root chakra is activated and the muscles in her pelvic floor tighten. Living in a range restricted by her bodily response to fear will continually limit a woman's ability to inhabit the fullness of her life or use her energy resources.

After witnessing the pelvic distress patterns arising post–September 11, I began to pay greater attention to the external events in the lives of my clients. I found that any significant life event registers its impact in a woman's root and pelvic floor, particularly when these events relate to loss, security, or transition. Experiences creating a root stress response for my clients have included a visit to the emergency room with an injured child, the death of a family member or friend, the loss of a longtime pet, a divorce or separation, moving from one location to another, and financial stress or employment changes for a woman or her partner.

A woman's body may also present in a state of high pelvic distress even though the traumatic experience initially triggering the stress response had occurred many years previously. Unless resolved with hands-on bodywork, distress in the root often continues to disrupt a woman's pelvic presence and energy flow.

In working with pelvic layers, I have seen distress patterns arise in women as they call to mind family members who suffered or died, such as in the Holocaust, or while acknowledging other profound wounds of their ancestors. Whether a woman experiences a traumatic event directly or carries the imprint from her lineage, the extent of its impact on her root depends upon receiving a core resolution that will restore her overall sense of well-being. Rather than focusing on the story of trauma, she can work to restore the energy flow that was disrupted.

The beauty of the pelvic bowl is that simply working with the body's response to trauma and stress may bring healing and restore a woman's access to her creative core. By addressing areas of energy blockage, a woman's inner range is no longer defined by these restrictions. With practice in restoring her root energy flow, a woman gains the ability to overcome the fear and resolve the trauma response that would otherwise block her full creative potential. She can process the energy of future stressful events with greater resources and deepen the root strength for herself and for all her creations.

## Move Beyond Fear

If you have experienced a profound loss or been attacked, emotionally or physically, you have reason to be afraid. But becoming frozen by this experience, within your energy and the fluidity of your body, alters your way of being. Freezing in fear does not allow for the dynamic response required in any future challenges. Succumbing to your fear also prevents you from transforming the pain of previous experiences into a source of strength.

Expect to encounter the constriction in your body, as a physical and energetic response to fear and at times of change, even when that change is desirable. Some causes of fear are imagined and some are real, but if you allow your body's response to fear to halt your progress, then your ability to embody your full creative range remains limited. Courage is continuing to invite challenge and change, and maintaining your core energy as strong and fluid, even in the presence of your deepest fear. Listen to the root voice saying, *This will never work* and *I don't think I can do this*, to find your capacity to move beyond fear. Think of someone who has done something bold with her life; notice how she transcended obstacles created by fear. Recognize the presence of fear as a signal that you are moving beyond past limits and expanding your range. By identifying your fear, you discover where to free your feminine potential.

### Exercise: Name Your Fear

Name your fear about your female body, femininity, or feminine power by finishing the statement "I am afraid of ..." Pay attention to the response in your pelvic energy as you contemplate your fear.

1. Reflection: Think about the significance of each fear that you named and what it calls your attention to. Examine the root of your fear and whether it arises from a lineage pattern, unacknowledged wound, unaddressed need, unclaimed potential,

or some other source. Change each statement of fear to "I want..." and fill in what you desire to reclaim.

2. Ritual: Ponder the desire conveyed by your fear with a spontaneous creation. Spend five minutes freewriting, drawing, dancing, or otherwise expressing the desire contained within your fear. When you are finished, notice your pelvic energy again. How has it changed? How has your relationship with fear changed?

*Women's Stories: Facing Fear in the Birth Process*

Stella came for pelvic work to assist her postpartum healing two months after delivering a baby. As she received the vaginal massage, she recalled the intense fear she experienced as her uterus dilated during childbirth. She said she had been calmly moving through labor when suddenly she became afraid. Stella felt that her body was "ripping apart," and this sensation made it very difficult for her to surrender into the expansion required for her daughter's birth.

A powerful opening occurs in the birth process. Stella wanted to retreat from the intensity of this physical and emotional experience. Her midwife looked directly into her eyes and held her hands, which kept Stella present with her body through each contraction. By feeling the sensations of her body, she focused less on her fear. Stella said that it felt as if her midwife was holding her, helping her to trust her body, so that her uterus was able to keep opening. When her daughter was born, having transcended her fear, Stella was ecstatic.

**Transform Your Fear**

To birth any creation or to change your creative range, you will face your fear of physical, creative, and emotional expansion. The root voice of fear is a potential ally for teaching you about opportunities for growth. Instead of turning away from fear, begin to notice and observe your response to it. Touch your root and notice how it tightens when you call your fear to mind. Then do a session of vaginal massage to clear the fear-based tension in your core. Teaching your body to soften even in the presence of alarm lessens fear's hold on you and keeps it from blocking your potential.

Pay attention to the response in your breath, energy, and thought patterns whenever your fear arises. Does your breathing become restricted when you think about a new possibility? Do you notice your energy freezing in reaction to fear? Take a breath to keep your energy moving, particularly in your root. Direct your breath toward your ovaries, inviting their healing warmth to flow through your center. Change the direction of your focus toward your desire rather than your fear. Envision yourself experiencing the joy and challenge in whatever presents itself to you.

As you listen to your root voice of fear, you will find your limits. Challenge these edges, and you will feel them shift. Use the resources of your pelvic bowl to encourage the flow of your creative energy. Keep expanding your self-concept to find your new edge. Trust the path that frees you from your fear, even when it is difficult.

I invite you to use a mantra or rhythmic chant when feeling afraid. Mantras assist the gathering of energy to support you in changing form. Repeat the following mantra, or one of your own, until your body softens or breath deepens.

> *I trust my body.*
> *I trust my path.*
> *I breathe my faith.*
> *I am not alone.*

Each time a fear arises, it is an opportunity to change your core structure to reflect expansion rather than limitation. When you feel the constriction response of fear in your body, you are close to the walls holding back your full creative flow. Listen to the wisdom and guidance present in your root voice of fear, but keep your energy fluid and moving to expand beyond these walls and find your true potential. Reflections on transforming your fear include:

How is fear restricting your radiance?
What will change by letting go of this fear?
How would you like to live more boldly?
How can you meet your fear with faith?

## Give Life to Your Creations

I am on a prayer walk. My friend is pregnant and bleeding. Knowing that she may miscarry, she has called me to her. Her house is just a few blocks from mine. It is a hot day, and I decide to walk and drum. I am walking and drumming my prayer for her and the soul of her child. I am thinking, as I walk, about a fall that I took with my newborn son and the thin line between life and death.

When my first son was born, my protective instincts rose up out of nowhere. I wanted to shield him from all harm. My ability to protect him had lasted for thirty-seven days when, with one slight misstep, I tripped and fell on the sidewalk. I still shudder when I recall the impact, the way we fell together, my baby's head hitting the concrete. An X-ray would later confirm my fears—my son had a skull fracture.

As women, we are creators. This is the truth of our wombs. As the givers of life, we long to keep our creations from harm and especially from death. Yet our creations have lives of their own. We long to protect them, and how we do so affects their ability to live.

The night I stayed in the hospital with my baby son, watching the rise and fall of his chest for any change in its steady rhythm, I learned another truth: I could not protect my son from his fate. By acting from fear and sheltering him from the hazards of living, I might restrict his potential. I would protect him best by offering my solid presence in whatever circumstances life might bring him. Trusting the workings of spirit in this way, I would let my son live his life to its full capacity.

In forming each creation, women must come to terms with the desire to hold on and the necessity of letting go. We feel a tension between creating something and surrendering to its unique path, and our intuitive drive to nurture prompts us to hold our creations close, but we must also give them to life. We close ourselves from the presence of life if we are too afraid of death. We limit our relationships with our creations if we are unable to let them go.

It is a test of our faith to allow each creation its process of living its own, independent life. Perhaps this is why Mary, mother of Jesus, is esteemed. She had the tremendous faith to stand by her son, even as she witnessed his fate. A mother must have courage to encourage (literally "give courage") to her children. We might model how focus and faith are healthy responses to fear, but this still does not give us control over the outcome of events. The best way of nurturing our creations, or ourselves, is to work with each growth experience with the intention of deepening our connection to spirit, rather than resisting or trying to shape the path that is unfolding. Surrendering to the flow of life while maintaining our conscious presence, we also receive its blessing.

Children grow, and our duty to them becomes more spiritual and less physical as they find their way into the world. This is true for all our creations. When we understand the creative process and match our energy to its natural progression, we have a purer relationship with what we have created. Rather than blocking the flow of life, our arms are free to applaud every step along the way. We become more available to embrace our children when they return, wounded by life's inevitable sorrows. We offer authentic protection, not restricting but celebrating the potential of each creative event in our lives. Open to this flow of life, we find our joy with each creation as well.

## Women's Stories: Completing a Birth Process

Tara came to see me a few weeks after the birth of her first child. She brought her baby to the appointment, and he was sleeping quietly in a baby carrier. Tara seemed a bit disoriented and expressed a sense of disconnect from her body. As I felt the energy in her pelvic bowl, I found that it still had the fullness of pregnancy. Tara had not completed the energetic release of birth energy from her womb.

I am trained in a process of bodywork created to resolve birth trauma in infants, pioneered by Dr. Sheila Murphy, a chiropractor and psychotherapist. I studied this holistic bodywork, designed to resolve the impact of trauma held in the body, with Dr. Murphy after the traumatic fall with my first son. When my one-month-old baby had been cleared to go home from the hospital, his cranial fracture was stable—but things still were not right. My son cried more readily, spitting up, though he had not done so before, and his little body felt rigid in my arms. We both held the impact of his fall, a tension in our bodies, until he received bodywork from Dr. Murphy.

In the first session with Dr. Murphy, my baby completely relaxed under her touch. He held her hands as if to say, "Thank you," and I cried tears of relief witnessing his response. Her work healed the trauma event for our family, and we received the additional blessing of Dr. Murphy's presence in our lives. I studied with her for two years and learned how to read and resolve trauma in infants' bodies. My new understanding of how trauma could impact the body honed my skills for working with the pelvic bowl in women.

Drawing on this trauma resolution experience, I sensed that the birth process for Tara and her baby had been interrupted in some way. I began to work on her pelvic bowl and invited her to connect with her womb, releasing any birth energy she might find. She began to focus her attention, and her pelvic bowl warmed with the energy of release. Then, all of a sudden, the energy stopped. I asked how she was doing, and Tara told me about her birthing experience: She had birthed at home and bled quite a bit afterward; the midwives were concerned about her bleeding, and Tara could feel the fear in the room. She brought all her focus to clamping down her womb in an effort to stop the bleeding. Instead of the natural release that accompanies a birth, Tara was still holding the birth energy in her body.

I encouraged Tara to recognize that she had made it to the other side of birthing; she was now six weeks postpartum, and her body could safely release its remaining birth energy. She began to breathe into her womb again, and her pelvis became warm from the uterine release. Then suddenly, the energy flow stopped again. I asked Tara what was happening, and she shared her fears with me. Having had two miscarriages prior to her baby's birth, she felt she had to hold on to this baby to keep from losing him. Even now, she was afraid to fully let go, fearing another loss.

I invited Tara to look over at her sleeping baby and recognize that he had also made it to the other side of the birth process. She turned toward him and began to cry. Seeing that he was indeed safely here with her she began to let go, releasing the energy from her core. A tremendous heat entered and then was released from her pelvic bowl. At the same time, Tara's baby began to stir, twisting his body and pushing his legs, as if moving down the birth canal. From my training with Dr. Murphy, I recognized these movements. However, I had never witnessed the relationship between an energy release from a woman's body and her baby's simultaneous response—their energy connecting to each other from across the room.

I lifted Tara's baby to her belly, where he continued to move, this time toward her breast. With our support, he latched on to his mother's nipple. Tara was laughing and crying; they also had been having difficulty with breastfeeding. The baby's mouth was wide on her nipple, and he was drinking her milk with the most solid latch yet.

A few weeks after working with Tara and her son, I was talking with a neighbor, a writer, about the connections between mothers and their children. He shared his experience that when his mother died a few years previously, he had received a burst of energy in his life. From my work with the pelvic bowl and from my knowledge of how energy comes through or is held back in the birth doorway, this exchange from mother to son made perfect sense. How much better, though, if women understood their potential to pass energy on to their children. Then from the very moment of birth, they could give their children the life force that belongs to them, receiving in return the invitation to witness the fullness of their child's life.

If you are a mother, imagine the creative energy of your womb going to each of your children, giving them their rightful life force energy. Mothering a child brings tremendous potential for growth, particularly if you are willing to examine your vulnerabilities in the mothering process. But giving attention to your own wounds related to mothering may stir feelings of regret. Rather than becoming stuck in the past, call your creative energy to the present so you may continue to evolve as a mother and creative woman, trusting the mothering path. Ponder the following questions for each of your children, even if they are grown:

What energy has my child always carried as a vital part of his or her being?

How can I encourage this energy flow in my child's life?
Do I have any regret regarding my mothering of this child?
How can I work with the energy of my regret to give more
   life force and support to my child?
What gifts have I given to my child?
What is my prayer for my child?
How can I live my truth so that I meet my child with joy?

Remember too that you are the child of your mother and father, a unique creation. Imagine receiving all your life force essence, from your own beginning, to energize your body and your being. Tapping into the energy of the earth (our original mother) by seeking the wild will also revitalize your energy, so take note of how you feel after spending time in a wild place.

Giving life to your creations also means trusting the creative process. Your creations blossom by virtue of the divine forces that transform seeds into plants that bear fruit. You may want to have a baby, a satisfying career, a connection to spirit, a stronger body, more access to your joy, a new relationship—but whatever you are creating, you must surrender your control. Choose your seeds and where to plant them, and then let go to spirit. If your creations are not taking shape in the way you desire, do not give up hope. If you want to grow corn, keep planting corn. Learn from each harvest cycle and from those who grow their gardens well. Apply what you know the next time you sow your seeds. The creative process is sacred and mystical. Ask for what you want—but make room for the mystery—and then see how your bounty is manifested.

## Create Pelvic Boundaries

Pelvic boundaries mark the sacred space where a woman gestates her creations. To do her creative work, and to delve into the intimate and vulnerable process of creating from her core, a woman needs these invisible demarcation lines declaring *This is mine* and *This is yours*. Boundaries are a set of internal needs and intuitive insights about a woman's personal and rightful space. They allow her to maintain her body and her energy as separate, and they give her the necessary privacy to be present with her own creative desires and relationship with spirit.

In the quiet of her center, with boundaries that keep the endless demands of the outer world at bay, a woman will hear the intuitive, inner voice that says, *This is your creative dream* or *Move in this direction*. Boundaries also surround the energetic space a woman holds, keeping her from feeling drained or intruded upon by another person's energy. They allow her to feel safe, and they serve as a container, meant to be filled with her own vital life force. Rather than rigid walls, healthy boundaries are flexible, able to change with each encounter and experience.

My clients are conscious and strong women, yet none have entered my office with clear pelvic boundaries. They may have surrendered their boundaries in response to an experience of pain or disrespect or simply inherited an expectation of creative or energetic compromise. Many women have survived various forms of violation to their female bodies and disregard for their feminine selves, and their boundaries are weakened as a result of these wounds. Instead of a solid energetic boundary around the body, and particularly around the pelvic bowl, women live with energetic holes that drain their creative energies and leave them less protected.

Even though pelvic boundaries govern the movement and usage of a woman's creative energy, most women are unaware of how these defining lines shape their creative lives. A woman's pelvic space is the rightful realm of what she chooses to nurture—both physically as she draws upon her root energy to tend to her children, produce creative work, or receive her partner in times of intimacy, and spiritually as she cultivates her own life as a creative being. But many others will desire to be held in her female energy system. A woman must be present in her pelvis and aware of her organ energy patterns to make conscious choices about what she takes into her sacred feminine space.

By studying the energy patterns of her body and learning where she disassociates or gives up her creative energy, a woman may reestablish and strengthen the boundaries that protect her space. Boundaries made with a woman's full energetic presence are strong and clear.

Robust pelvic boundaries serve your well-being as a woman, as they allow you to claim your creative and nurturing female energy for yourself and your desires. By establishing these boundaries, you are able to meet others more directly and receive the energy of your choosing. You are able to sustain closer and more intimate relationships with those you love, without compromising your needs or giving up your ground.

The boundaries of the pelvic space are diminished in their strength when you lose the grounding focus available in your root. As a child, you may have given up your feminine ground because others required it, but as a grown woman you relinquish your claim to this space because you are unaware of the energy patterns in your core. Your body and the gestational space for your creations are unprotected in the absence of clear pelvic boundaries. Increase your energetic presence in your root, and you will be more grounded. You will define your creative space whether in the midst of a challenging situation or in working on one of your creations. Ask yourself these questions to assess your boundary needs:

How do you define your creative space?
When have you noticed yourself feeling compromised or
     taking in unwanted emotional or other energy?
What do you need to maintain your sense of self and state
     of well-being?
What does this boundary express about you?

When you honor the boundaries of another person, you come to know them more intimately. As you honor the boundaries you establish for yourself, you come to know and trust yourself as well. As a female, you may have learned to place the needs of others first, but in doing so you dishonor yourself and maintain the sense that your feminine energy is not your own. Clear energetic boundaries will ensure that, even amid the intensity of taking care of a child or working in a busy professional role, there is always room to replenish and respond to the promptings of your creative core. Your vital feminine self will be more likely to emerge when you create and honor boundaries.

### Women's Stories: Finding Her Creative Ground

Paula came to my office to strengthen her core muscles and root connection. She mentioned feeling very disconnected from her pelvis and had difficulty engaging with several facets of her life. As I began to work on her root muscles, the tension they contained was resistant to any change, and her vital energy was almost completely blocked. I asked her how she felt about being female. She laughed, but there was also pain in her voice as she told me that her father had not wanted any daughters and her mother had low self-esteem. Paula had spent many years with a counselor working on her own self-esteem issues.

As I sat with Paula, I could sense the lack of value in her core by the absence of her own awareness. She had abandoned her root, a part of her body that defined her as female, perhaps in response to the lack of value she experienced in her family. She had given up her own creative ground, knowing she had disconnected from her feminine organs, but not realizing that by doing so she had internalized the pattern of devaluing women in her family.

I encouraged Paula to bring her breath and internal awareness back to her pelvic bowl to restore her creative presence and energetic flow. The muscles of her root became very hot as the energy and blood began to move. After a few minutes, the heat dispersed and the tension in her core released. It was a simple process to help Paula reconnect, and yet until a woman addresses her core energy patterns, she will continue to lose the vital energy of her creative center.

Bringing awareness back to her pelvic bowl on a regular basis may require Paula to address, with a counselor or a ritual, the feelings of shame and grief from her past wounding. But each wave of emotional energy that she integrates will assist her in changing her core patterns. Rather than avoiding her root because her family did not know how to honor women (likely due to their own feminine wounding), she can set new pelvic boundaries that convey her worth: *women are precious*; *women are strong*; *my pelvis is sacred*. With energetic boundaries that honor her core, Paula will be able to inhabit her creative ground and reengage with life from her center.

## Ovarian Energy and Pelvic Boundaries

Balanced ovarian energy is essential for maintaining a woman's pelvic boundaries. After learning about her pelvic boundaries, a client shared her experience of using her ovarian energy. She had noticed that when she was in a public space and was made uncomfortable by someone, bringing awareness to both ovaries dissipated her sense of vulnerability. By breathing toward the ovaries and strengthening the energy of her pelvic presence, a woman is able to stay centered and prevent herself from receiving unwanted energy, either from strangers or even challenging situations with loved ones. When a woman maintains her conscious presence in the energy of her root, she creates an extremely effective pelvic energetic boundary.

To strengthen your pelvic boundaries, use the following exercise for balancing ovarian energy. Examine your ovarian patterns and pay attention to when or how you lose your pelvic boundaries. Identify any changes you desire to make in the boundaries of your pelvic bowl by noticing how you receive or use creative energy.

### Exercise: Creating Pelvic Boundaries

Find a comfortable position. It is ideal to sit directly on the ground during this exercise. Read the exercise through first, and then close your eyes to begin.

1. Guide your attention internally to your pelvic space. What are the boundaries that define this space? What is the quality of your energy or radiance in your center?

2. Where do you lose touch with the boundaries of your pelvic space? Recall an experience that felt invasive to you and notice what happens to your pelvic presence.

3. Bring your focus to the left ovary, a place midway between your pubic bone and the top left side of your pelvis. Inhale and draw the energy from the earth up your left leg and into the left pelvis and ovary. As you exhale, move the energy into your womb and then down again into the earth. Shift your weight to the left side and feel the solid edges of the physical and energetic boundary of the left half of your pelvic bowl. Continue sensing and visualizing the energy flow between your left ovary and the earth, following your breath for ten repetitions or as long as feels necessary.

4. Bring your focus to the right ovary, a place midway between your pubic bone and the top right side of your pelvis. With an inhalation, draw the energy from the earth up your right leg and into the right pelvis and ovary. As you exhale, move

the energy into your womb and then down into the earth. Shift your weight to the right side and feel the solid edges of the physical and energetic boundary of the right half of your pelvic bowl. Continue sensing and visualizing the energy flow between your right ovary and the earth, following your breath for ten repetitions or as long as feels necessary.

5. Return your attention to the center of your pelvic space. Notice what has changed. Is your ovarian energy more balanced? Do you have a more equal sense of warmth in the left and right sides of your pelvis? Notice the multidimensional aspects of your pelvic bowl, the way that energy can radiate in all directions.

6. Imagine the same invasive experience that you envisioned previously. What happens to your pelvic energy? Are you able to maintain your pelvic presence? If so, you increased your ability to hold your pelvic boundaries. If not, read chapter 4 and learn how to gather more of your ovarian energy; then repeat this exercise. What further actions will strengthen your claim to this space?

7. Bring your visualization to a close. Offer thanks for your feminine ground, your very own place for cultivating and protecting your creative essence.

## Claim Your Creative Space

With intact pelvic boundaries, you are better able to claim your creative space. Look for where you have given up your creative ground and learn how to reestablish your core energetic boundaries. Some women claim their creative energy in work but not in the home. Others forgo the energy available to them in the womb space if they have not carried a child there. Pain, infertility, abuse, dysfunctional lineage patterns, or other pelvic wounds may have caused you to forget regions of your pelvic bowl. Reclaim your ground in these places most of all.

The root of the body gives a woman many signals before she loses her pelvic boundaries and begins to relinquish her energetic space. However, she must be present in the pelvic bowl to notice the signs of physical tension or energy stagnation that notify her of her need to restate her claim to her core or take a break to recover her center.

If a woman finds herself repeatedly challenged to maintain pelvic boundaries during a specific circumstance, I invite her to call this situation to mind while staying aware of her pelvic bowl. Each time she loses her focus, she has lost her pelvic boundaries; she must regain her pelvic presence by connecting to her root with her breath and internal vision. She practices this process of reconnection until she feels ready to hold her internal focus, even when faced directly with the person or situation that challenges her.

Maintaining pelvic presence creates such firm boundaries that a woman may experience conflict with anyone who resists them. However, if she stands her ground, she will find that pelvic boundaries ultimately offer a deeper connection with those who respect her stance and greater protection from those who do not. Over time, people around her will respond to her steady root presence. The energy in her relationships will begin to move more sustainably. The way that she connects with others will evolve, and the tension in her core is released. Everyone breathes more easily, able to inhabit their rightful place.

When you claim your space in the root of your body, you can also claim your space in the outer world. Look within your pelvic bowl and find the attitudes, emotions, and energies that diminish your vitality. Clarify the values that honor your womanhood and clear anything else from your core. Focus on the creations that fuel your joy. Listen from your root, and you will know which relationships and habits to change or renegotiate. Reflections on claiming your creative space include:

Where do you give up your ground?

When do you worry instead of trusting the creative movement at hand?

When do you take in the energy of a stressful encounter instead of holding joy in your core?

Where do you desire to change the boundaries that define your feminine range?

## Do Your Lineage Work

As I teach women to engage the root of the female body, I regularly encounter patterns in lineage or energy that have been passed down and still perpetuate in families, so I have come to recognize the profound importance of lineage work. For women to create firm pelvic boundaries and renegotiate the lines that define their creative potential, they must reexamine the habitual and learned patterns regarding their female energy. Only by doing their lineage work to transform these inherited and often unconscious patterns are women able to clarify and strengthen their presence in their bodies and gain access to their full wild-feminine range. The information that I share regarding lineage energy is derived from my work in the root of the female body to change core patterns and restore or enhance core energy flow.

I learned about the lineage patterns in my own body by exploring the energy of my root. One day, while meditating on the grief in my womb that accompanied my miscarriage, my paternal grandmother came to mind. She had lost her fourth baby near term.

This child, my grandmother's last son, was stillborn—my father's little brother. I saw an image of this baby in my meditation, and I pondered my grandmother's experience of loss. With three boys to mother already, how did she mourn the death of her youngest son? I said a prayer for her and her baby, as well as for my father—who was just a toddler at the time—and his two older brothers.

After my meditation, I telephoned my father and suggested we travel to visit my grandmother. She was quite elderly and living in a care facility, having been uncommunicative for years. Because I lived across the country, I had not seen or talked to her since long before my first son was born. My father agreed, and we made arrangements for our trip.

That night, I pulled back the covers to my bed. An image of my grandmother flashed into my mind. She was in her bed and there was light all around her. I was standing at the foot of her bed, with my young son in my arms. I had only one child at the time and was uncertain about taking him on a cross-country trip. When I saw this image in my mind, I took it as a sign that I should take my son to see my grandmother, his great-grandmother. I looked at my son, asleep in my bed, and laid down next to him.

I do not remember falling asleep, but I was dreaming when the phone rang. I thought it was still night, but when I lifted my head from the pillow, I saw the dawn sky just outside my window. From the dry tone of my father's voice on the phone, I knew that my grandmother had died.

I believe my grandmother was waiting to die. The timing of her death that night, just after my father and I made our travel plans, seemed confirmation. It was as if she had held on to life until certain that her connection with us was not lost. For many years, I had thought of her as gone, dead already—but she was not. When she died just as I began to remember her, I understood the depth of our bond.

My father and I still traveled to see her, but we came instead for her funeral. Though she had died, I remembered my vision of her on the eve of her death and felt the warmth of her spirit. Listening to the grief of my miscarriage and delving into the emotional depths of my womb allowed me to hear her and connect with my lineage. Still, I wished I had not stayed away from her so long. Given the timing of my grandmother's death, I paid closer attention to the energy of my womb and the way it directed my focus to certain aspects of my lineage.

Meditating on my womb, I wondered about forgotten members of my maternal ancestry. My maternal grandparents, who were always in my life, responded to my requests for family knowledge with pictures of people I had never seen before. Spending time with these photos and researching the lands where these ancestors had lived brought a sense of warmth and energy to my body. I was particularly drawn to my grandfather's grandmother, Matilda, whose energy I could feel in a line of women behind me. When I received a photo of her holding my great-grandmother on her lap, I felt an immediate rise of joy. I learned that Matilda, born in Sweden, sailed to the United States from Norway, and I began to see her in my dreams. Seeing her allowed me to understand the thread of lineage that I carry in my hands and in my healing practice.

In various cultures and eras, ancestors have been ritually honored. We can likewise honor our own ancestors. We honor them for their importance in our lives and their imprints in our bodies. By acknowledging them and mourning their sacrifices, we discover the gifts of our lineage. We can receive ancestral wisdom and support, and the energetic strength of the lines that we carry, when we pay homage to these people who came before us. Each step taken by one of our ancestors has prepared the way for us to be here, just as our steps now prepare the way for our descendants. When we give thoughtful regard to our place in our lineage, we understand the undercurrent of energy that gives expression to our lives.

## Research Your Lineage: Find Your Threads

The first step in remembering your ancestors is to research your lineage and find your personal connection to it, your own lineage threads. Learn about the countries or read the works of writers from the lands of your ancestors. Speak with the elders in your family or anyone who has experience with the time and place of your research. Listen to their stories, both for what is said and for what remains unsaid. Remember whether most of your ancestors were immigrants or whether they lived for many generations in one place. Acknowledge their experiences of loss—whether of children who died or of families separated by distance and time.

If you have a lineage tree, try to fill in missing names or other identifying information. Look for patterns such as certain birthdays, careers, or patterns in gender and number of children (I have three sons and my father and maternal grandfather each had two brothers). Trace your maternal and paternal lines. Notice how the flow of information on paper represents the flow of these energy lines in your body and your life.

Some lineage threads may be obvious—for example, a passion for gardening that arises from a family of farmers or a medical profession in a family of doctors or healers. Others you may never know directly or you may discover by accident. I adore hats and am known for wearing them, yet I was still surprised to learn that one of my great-grandmothers was a hatmaker. Finding these threads and cultivating them will assist the flow of lineage energy in your body, which relates to your purposeful work in life. I carry a spiritual thread arising from many sources: land-based spiritual connections, Mormon pioneers, and my paternal grandfather who was a preacher. I strengthen the flow of this thread by honoring many different spiritual practices and having a daily communion with spirit, which rejuvenates my creative energy and serves my work as both a mother and a healer.

Together, the members of a lineage make a great tapestry, a grand weaving of many lives; individually, the members carry the threads of a lineage in their own way. Identifying your own threads in this tapestry will enhance your lineage flow. By studying your family line or following the passions that enliven your own creative energy, you will find your lineage threads. Remember that these threads belong to a lineage whose collective energy you tap when doing your creative work. Pay particular attention to the family lines that intrigue you—specific cultures, rituals, professions, land-scapes, or other inspirations that resonate in your core. Reflect on the following questions to better understand your lineage.

What traits or tendencies do you notice in yourself that reflect the lineage you carry?

Which parts of your lineage do you naturally connect with? What gift or lesson does this bring to your life?

Which parts of your lineage do you avoid or have limited information about? What do you need to address in these cases to restore this thread of your lineage?

Gather with family for a meal or a holiday and observe the line-age patterns that each of you carries. Ponder your roles in the family—the storyteller, the caretaker, the one who forges new ground and brings fresh inspiration. When you take time to reflect on your place in a lineage, you recover your ancestral energy and a vital link to the energy resources, built over many generations, that will serve your work in the present.

## Awaken the Cellular Memory of Lineage

In working with the energy of the body, I have found that an essen-tial part of lineage work is awakening the cellular memory of lineage through the senses of taste, sight, and sound. It also happens to be the most enjoyable part of lineage work. I was researching a line of my ancestors who came from Scotland when I happened to pass by a Scottish store one day. I had driven the same way many times, but I had never noticed this shop. I entered and was immedi-ately immersed in all things Scottish. I leafed through pictures of Scotland, pored over a map of the old regions that denoted various family clans, and found my great-grandfather's regional clan and tartan (a plaid scarf with his family's specific color and print pattern). I sampled some Scottish cookies and, eyeing the round metal flasks in a glass case, wondered if this was where my taste for whiskey had come from.

Another time, I was visiting a friend and happened upon a regional Scandinavian festival which came from the same location as another branch of my ancestors. I have always loved woolen shawls and leather boots and was surprised to see many of them in this festival. One booth had a few antique wool blankets woven in natural dyes; looking at the patterns of these blankets and running my fingers over the soft weavings engaged my senses in a deep and familiar way. This same booth also had a pair of old leather boots that looked almost the same as the pair I was wearing. I wandered the aisles, observing my joyful response—the signs of my own lineage thread coming to life.

The cellular memories you carry are often awakened through the senses. The lineage memory evoked by the senses explains how a picture of an ancestral homeland or a family heirloom held in the hand can induce an emotional response, even when its particular stories are unknown. If you are adopted, you draw energy from the ancestors of your adoptive family as well as those of your birth family. Any place that the lineage members or stories are unknown, you may do research on cultures of the world that seem to call your attention. You may have a thread of lineage from one of these places, and the lineage energy will flow more freely in your life once you awaken the sensory memory of your cells. Immerse yourself in the tastes, colors, stories, symbols, and textures of a given people and place.

Wherever your lineage is unknown or there are gaps in your knowledge, meditate on your womb space. The wordless knowledge here will provide what is needed if you sit and ask for it. The stories of your ancestors are not lost; you will find them humming in your bones. The following exercise may assist you.

*Exercise: Lineage Meditation*

1. Bring awareness to your womb, the center of your pelvic space. When you feel that all your attention is here, begin to sense the energy that sits behind you, just to the left and right of your pelvic bowl. This is the energy of your lineage. From working with women's bodies, I have observed the energy of the maternal line on the left and of the paternal line on the right. Imagine your mother and her lineage sitting behind you on the left side, your father and his lineage sitting behind you on the right, if this feels true for you.

2. Sense the quality of each energy line. Recognize that these are formed by the many branches that extend behind you as your lineage tree. Just as the leaves on a tree draw energy from the sun and channel that energy into the rest of the tree, so you draw upon these ancient branches for your own energy flow. When the energy of your lineage is supporting your life, it will feel like a strong current flowing from all these branches into your body, magnifying your creative potential.

3. The mother and father lines represent the energy of your ancestors, which you carry on as part of your lineage pattern. Notice where the energy is clear and strong, overflowing or underflowing. Sense whether the energy of your lineage comes together with resistance or ease. Ask your body what is needed to support your lineage energy flow. Whatever you observe is helpful in clarifying or transforming your lineage patterns.

4. Recognize that this energy of your lineage represents the lives of many individuals, most of whom no longer walk the earth. Take a moment to acknowledge and honor them.

Imagine your full lineage tree and notice if a particular branch calls your attention.

5. Recognize that a tree also extends in front of you, representing the energy of those who will descend from you or other family members. Your creative seeds extend from here as well. Contemplate the energy you are presently carrying forward, the offerings for your lineage.

6. Bring your meditation to a close with gratitude and awareness for your essential place in your lineage.

*Note: When people are adopted, they can still attune themselves to the energy of these mother and father lines. Tapping into the lineage energy that flows through the body can be healing when the physical lines have been disrupted. Some of my clients who were adopted as children have told me they feel the energy of their adoptive parents flowing on either side of the energy of their birth parents. This type of combined energy is similar to that found in tribal societies, where many adults surround and care for each child. In a similar fashion, a woman may draw upon the support of people who, although unrelated to her, have become part of her lineage fabric through their important caretaking roles in her life.*

## Balance the Flow of Your Mother and Father Lines

Certain lines of your lineage will speak to you, but be sure to draw from both your mother and father lines. Balance the ancestral energy in your core. On one side of my family, I have immigrants and pioneers—people who seek adventure and forge trails. On the other side, I come from people who lived their whole lives in one place, generations of people tending the same ground. Out of balance, these opposing energies would be at odds in my center.

Woven together, they provide both the creative initiative I use to discover new ground and the stability to sustain my creations. I call to mind the large, hand-carved wooden bowl in my kitchen, and with it the stable energy of my father line, as a reminder to cook and nourish myself even when following my creative passions. I go to the ocean and make a fire, stirring the energy of my mother line, whenever I need fresh inspiration in my life.

Your female body will direct you to the regions of your lineage that require attention in order to restore the energy flow of your lines. For example, if the lineage energy is strong on the right side but weak on the left, look to the lineage of your mother. Connect to your maternal lineage with more intention or seek to uncover the blockages that limit your access. If, instead, you have a history of right-sided body issues, work with the energy patterns of your father line.

Sometimes there is a conflict between the lineages themselves, resulting from familial, cultural, or other differences. Work with these energies in your body to promote peace and harmony in your center. Call on the playful and productive masculine energies (and heal the negative masculine forms that operate through aggression and domination) that arise from both sides of your lineage to reinspire your own masculine nature; call on the nurturing and intuitive feminine energies (and heal patterns of victimization that signal a disempowered feminine) from both sides of your lineage to reinspire your own feminine nature. When the energies of both lines are running strongly and blending in your core, you can draw from them to support and invigorate your body and your daily life. Reflections regarding balancing the flow of your lines include:

What patterns do you notice in your mother and father lines?

Are there any points of tension in these lines or within your body?

What traits of each line might be beneficial in your life? How can you balance and draw upon these energies?

*Women's Stories: Rediscovering Her Father Line*

Celia came for pelvic work to renew her vital energy. She felt drained and had difficulty finishing her daily tasks in her home. With the postpartum demands on her body from a recent childbirth, she was in need of pelvic rebalancing. However, we also discovered a familial pattern that was inhibiting her female energy system from replenishing itself.

As I assessed Celia's pelvic patterns, I noticed that the majority of her pelvic strength was on the left side and she had little awareness or ability to engage her muscles on the right side. When I asked her to focus her attention on the pelvic space, she noticed that she naturally gravitated to the left and avoided the right side of her pelvis.

In my work with clients, I listen to many women tell their stories. When they are talking about issues regarding their mother, they generally tend to gesture to the left. When they are talking about their father, they tend to gesture to the right. Likewise, when I am working in the pelvic space and a woman is talking about her mother or her mother's family, the left pelvic muscles often tense or move in some way. When a woman is talking about her father or her father's family, the right side of the pelvis responds.

Having seen mother and father lineage patterns in the bodies of many women, and knowing the ways that our bodies organize energy imprints and flow, I understand the potential in the female body. Family history is highly subjective, based on the stories that are told. Even the stories themselves require interpretation, as each contains subtle nuances that are rarely understood unless one has lived in the fabric of their embrace.

So much of the information that women need in order to heal family patterns is either unspoken or unknown. The female body offers each woman guidance to the imprints of her familial energetic patterns. Each woman needs to learn to read the signs, and as a result, she will find the potential places for focused healing work and the ways in which to reclaim what was lost.

With Celia, I inquired about her connection with her father line because her pelvic presence was diminished on the right side. She told me that her father was not a part of her life, that he had left the family when she was nine years old and died three years later. Celia wanted to reconnect with his essence and this part of her lineage, particularly after having children, but she did not know how to do so, since her father had died.

Focusing on the right side of her pelvic bowl, Celia thought about her father and the pain that he carried from his own wounds that caused him to be so absent. I asked her to focus on the sensations in her pelvis, and she noticed a profound tension on the right, a sense of closing in. I encouraged her to bring breath to this space. With focused breathing, the energy began to change. Celia observed the change in her body, and her eyes filled with tears. She recognized how much she longed for the support of her father's presence in her life and how much weight she had carried on her own. Acknowledging these burdens allowed a release of the tension, and her pelvic bowl became warmer and filled with light.

Celia had a box of her father's things, old photos of him, and a passion for cooking that he also shared. By looking to each of these for her connection with her father, she could remember his essence. Cooking with him in mind, placing a photo of him on the wall, and responding to his memory in other ways would all revive the energy of his presence in her life. Remembering that her body was a direct link to her

father's essence, Celia could restore the flow of energy that
was her rightful inheritance. Reconnecting with these aspects
of her father increased her access to the imprint of his lineage
energy in her body and supported a greater flow of this masculine energy for reenergizing her life.

## Acknowledge the Wounds of Your Lineage

When you pay attention to your ancestry, you will encounter the
wounds of your lineage. These are the unmourned losses, unrealized
dreams, and other hurts suffered by your ancestors. These lineage
wounds tend to trap energy and have untold and diverse effects on
each member of a lineage. Acknowledging the pain of your ancestors, and allowing the blocked energy to release with a ritual or
meditation on the pelvic bowl, frees this energetic burden and
allows you to reclaim vital parts of your heritage and lineage
energy flow. The key to moving the lineage energy that was previously blocked is to focus on a healing movement to restore what
was lost (and to stay in the present moment by feeling the sensations in your body). Do this rather than focusing on the trauma
event itself.

I discovered in my own lineage that my great-grandfather had
remarried a few months after my great-grandmother died. His
daughter, my grandmother, never accepted his second wife, and
there was tension between the two women, even after his death.
In researching this line, I learned that my great-grandfather
was buried a few miles from my home and my step-great-
grandmother, Addie, lay buried next to him. One blustery day
I made the journey to these grave sites, bringing flowers for
Addie and scotch liquor to pour on the ground to honor my
great-grandfather's Scottish origins. I also pondered the loss
my grandmother must have felt after her own mother died and
her father moved on. I was making peace, intending to clear
the energy of this old wound. The air was bright and fresh on

the hillside where they lay. I felt giddy as I sat under the pine tree near their graves, perhaps receiving the inspiration of a newly freed lineage energy.

When you step into a role that echoes the lives of your ancestors, you activate lineage patterns in a purposeful manner for continuing the evolution and generational work related to a particular lineage thread. For example, when you get married, become a mother, or step into a professional role similar to that of your predecessors, the lineage energy in your body responds. Wound patterns can be activated as well; for example, if you have a miscarriage or experience a violation or loss that was similar to one experienced by your ancestors, you may feel the loss more deeply because it stirs the losses of your lineage. Likewise, any healing or resolution that you experience may free the older wound energy in unexpected ways. Focus on restoring balance in your pelvic bowl and on reclaiming the feminine and masculine aspects of your creative energy to recover your rightful range and send a healing wave down your mother and father lines. Reflections to help you acknowledge the wounds of your lineage include:

Where did the women and men of your lineage give up their ground?

How is this affecting your own core energy patterns?

What roles or wounds in your own life reflect issues from the past?

How are your lineage threads related to these roles or wound patterns?

## Patterns of Feminine Wounding

The defined range of the feminine is often passed along through lineage patterns. Study the patterns in your family, and you may be further inspired to challenge the undercurrents restricting your expression of the feminine.

By noticing the echo of feminine wounding in your body or present life, you can address the aspects of feminine identity that were restricted for your ancestors. When you work with these wounds in your core, you access the root medicine that brings true transformation. That transformation in your center frees your creative essence and the energy resources for your future creations. Look for patterns of wounding regarding the aspects of feminine identity that were hurtful for both women and men, as both genders have suffered from the degradation of the feminine. Reflections regarding feminine wounding and your lineage include:

How was femininity defined and perceived in your family?
What roles were available to women? How did they feel about these roles?
How were men blocked or accepted in expressing their emotions, creativity, and other feminine aspects?
Which men and women broke out of the family mold to create something new?

## Change the Flow of Your Lineage Lines

The wounds of a lineage and the flow of your lineage energy can be transformed in many ways. Even if the specific wounds are unknown, you can still reach out to the lineage and encourage a healthy movement of lineage energy. Tending a gravesite, spending time in meditation or prayer while remembering the life and challenges of a particular ancestor, or creating a ritual will honor and acknowledge a family line. The spiritual practices, harvest celebrations, and other traditions of your ancestors that have been done repeatedly over time contain energy resources for you, so reviving and renewing these traditions will activate this energy in your life. Making a piece of art, researching your family history, traveling to the land of your ancestors, or telling your children a story about their lineage are all ways to reconnect with your ancestors and receive their ancient energy into your life. Use the following ideas to assist your lineage work:

### Exercise: Healing Actions for Your Lineage

1. Patterns of disconnect: Restore the flow of your lineage in any place of disconnect by doing research, finding photos, listening to stories, meditating on your pelvic bowl, awakening the cellular memory of cultures and landscapes through your senses, and reviving the rituals and traditions of your lineage.

2. Patterns of loss: When you encounter a lineage loss, do a grief ritual, light a candle, or plant a flower to acknowledge and move the energy of loss. Restore the energy flow in the place of loss.

3. Restricted lineage roles: When you discover a place of restriction in the lines (for example, women can only be in the home, men must earn the money, or everyone in this family line is an alcoholic) gather some art materials and use the particular restriction as a theme to inspire your creative expression. See what you uncover in the process.

4. Creative range limitations: Directly challenge the defining lines and energy of lineage patterns that limit your creative range. For example, if your mother worked tirelessly while nurturing others, take breaks to rest and drink a cup of tea (or otherwise nurture yourself) in the midst of your daily life as a mother or other creative woman.

5. Boundary and other violations: If you know about or discover past violations to members of your lineage, heal

these wounds by addressing unconscious agreements about giving up your ground and strengthening the boundaries of your own pelvic bowl. Taking up your rightful space will bring healing and may inspire further work or ritual to call back whatever else may have been previously lost.

6. Devaluing of the feminine: Restore the flow of the feminine for your lineage by doing your own root work to nourish and honor your core, following your internal rhythms, and giving expression to your creative life. Revive an empowered masculine that protects, values, and aligns with the feminine.

7. Unrealized dreams: Remember the early deaths or other unrealized potentials of your lineage by taking time to plant your own creative seeds and nurturing them until they bear fruit. Celebrate your harvest and share the bounty with the spirits of your ancestors.

Whenever you experience a depth of emotion regarding your womanhood, particularly when it seems out of proportion to your present situation, you may be grappling with a lineage pattern representing generations of shame or disregard of the feminine. As you access the emotions connecting you to a lineage wound, you will move the energy blockages in your core. Underneath this energy of previously unexpressed feelings, you will find the gifts that are carried in your family lines.

Rather than disconnecting from the painful aspects of your lineage, create a ritual to honor your ancestors and acknowledge or move the energy imprint of their pain. Ask for the support of your ancestors in transforming the legacy of your lineage. Each family member carries a piece of the lineage in his or her own way, uniquely expanding the potential for healing. Notice the echo of lineage wounds in yourself by reflecting on the following:

What patterns do you notice in your lineage regarding feminine power, creativity, personal expression, and the female body?

How are you currently carrying the feminine (and masculine) wounds of your lineage?

What action will address one aspect of these wounds?

How can you receive a greater flow of energy from your lineage lines?

Take time to integrate each piece of lineage work to avoid being overwhelmed by the energy released. Gather your resources—family, friends, practitioners, the transformative capacity of your pelvic bowl, ritual practices, and prayers—to assist with the assimilation process. Consider the wounds you carry as source material for cultivating your creations, rather than as items to discard. Immerse yourself in a piece of lineage work, and then do an activity that lightens your mood. Focus on each step of the path rather than striving for a certain outcome; this will make the process of lineage work more sustainable. Invite along the playful essence of your wild feminine to bring a sense of delight as you do your lineage work and broaden your creative range.

## Expand Your Creative Range

The way a woman uses her creative essence defines her creative range. Many individuals inform a woman's creative capacity, and mothers have the earliest influence on the shape of this range and perspective of what is possible. Whether a mother tried to shield or support a child faced with pain or loss affects that grown child's ability to take creative risks. Whether a mother celebrated, ignored, or competed with her child's creations affects whether a child will learn to direct or dim her radiance. Where a mother feels a scarcity on some level, she often holds her own child back. By exploring the lines that define—and particularly that limit—her self-expression, each woman discovers her inheritance and the ability to reshape her creative range.

A tension arises in anyone working at her creative edge, whether nurturing a child or taking risks as an artist. As one of your mother's bodily creations, your comfort with this tension and overall creative vitality are initially governed by your mother's energetic capacity. As a grown woman, your creative center lies in your female body. Your root conveys your relationship with expression: whether you tend to hold yourself back or let yourself go. By examining and altering your patterns of energy and stretching beyond the edge of your inherited range, you will increase your creative flow.

Reflect on your mother, on her relationship with creativity, and on how it felt to be one of her creations. Know that any disappointments you carry are simply opportunities to reclaim your creative essence. If you do not know your mother, look to the patterns of using creative energy in your life. In the deep core patterns, you will discover your mother and the creative essence that now belongs to you. By working with these lines that define your creative capacity, you begin to reshape and expand your creative range. Reflections about expanding your creative range include:

How does your creative life reflect your creative range?

What did you learn about creativity from your mother? From your father?

How might you celebrate yourself as a creation?

How would you like to take a creative risk or expand your creative range?

## Recognize Your Own Resistance to Change

In building new patterns in your body and creative energy flow, you will encounter your own resistance to change. We resist change because old patterns are familiar, even if they are self-limiting or dysfunctional. It is easier to follow well-worn tracks than it is to forge a new path.

Resistance is manifested in the mind through patterns of avoidance or excuse making. It can be emotional, existing in patterns of numbness, explosive emotions, or denial of feelings, and it can also be expressed through patterns of disconnection and disrespect. Resistance can be physical as well, manifesting as patterns of tension and held energy in the muscles and organs of the body. Resistance is a density in the energy, so focusing your breath toward any places of holding or tension in your body will disperse the density and assist the energy flow, often diffusing your reactive response as well as helping to shift the underlying energy pattern.

In my work with women, I encourage them to address their resistance on all levels: tension in the body, blocks in the energy flow, emotional holding patterns, and limited modes of being. Often, when you encounter a strong sense of resistance in your core, you are also close to a breakthrough. Slow yourself down and pay attention to the sensations of your body. Rather than reacting to the resistance, find an engaged and curious response. Explore the edge marked by fear or rage, the defining lines that restrict your creative flow. Take a deep breath, focus on your root, let the energy soften and move, and expand into the fullness of your wild feminine range.

## Women's Stories: Celebrating the Wild

Amelia came for pelvic care to address a tight knot in the muscles on the right side of her vaginal opening. I began with massage to this region but found that her body was unresponsive, so I asked her to concentrate on the area of tension and describe her sensations.

Amelia noticed that her mind resisted her attempts to focus on the right side, but she continued to pay attention to her body, and she realized that her right ovary felt hardened and tightly wound. The longer she held her focus on the right side, the more her sense of internal resistance increased. When I asked what she was resisting, she paused and said that her primary challenge related to her son. They were frequently in conflict—her son was "stubborn and willful," just as her own father had described her. Amelia had had a distant relationship with her father, and she was afraid of having the same relationship problems with her son.

I encouraged her to pay attention to the resistance in her body. In doing so, she realized that she had a wall of tension and worry in her core about repeating her family pattern with her son. I invited Amelia to observe the physical sensation of resistance in her body. Just by acknowledging her fears and internal tension regarding her son, her body began to change. The region near the right ovary became extremely hot, releasing the energy, and I was able to begin working with the tension in her right pelvis.

I worked on the physical tension in Amelia's core and encouraged her to breathe toward any resistance she found. As we finished the session, Amelia told me she had a new perspective. Her father used to refer to her wildness in exasperation, like a wild horse in need of control. Amelia felt that her body's tension was related to these early attempts to control her expressive spirit. She also realized that her ex-husband had resisted her expansive nature as well. Attending to her center, she recognized a pattern in her relationship with males, but underlying this pattern, she saw that the early pattern of discord with her father had been internalized into a rejection of part of herself. By working with this internalized pattern, she felt certain that it would transform her way of relating to her son.

As she breathed into the tension in her body, Amelia could feel herself release some of this resistance. Now that she felt a greater sense of freedom in her body, she allowed herself to reconnect with her own wildness—she decided to stop resisting her young, wild self and let go of the negative associations that her father had imposed upon her. Imagining instead the strength and passion of a wild horse, Amelia was inspired to celebrate, rather than resist, the wildness in herself. Reintegrating this part of herself, she saw a new path for herself and her son.

## Renegotiate Unconscious Agreements

Agreements are the internal rules that inform your behavior, communication patterns, and interactions with others as well as the expectations you place upon yourself. They are a form of boundaries: defining lines that must be addressed to expand your range of feminine expression. Whether maintained by actions or held as beliefs, these agreements give meaning and structure to your life. They influence your sense of possibility, self-perspective, partnerships, and creative essence in a multitude of ways.

Unconscious agreements are the unspoken, often unacknowledged, rules governing your creative energy and capacity to create. They impact the development of your feminine identity through body beliefs, gender roles, family structures, intimate relationships, and cultural attitudes. Unconscious agreements impact your ability to maintain your boundaries and claim what is yours. They are unconscious because we often inherit and grow up with these agreements; so closely is our own essence entwined with them that we are largely unaware that these agreements are optional—to be maintained or renegotiated as we desire.

Unconscious agreements require renegotiation when they limit you or aspects of your personal expression, sense of power, self-worth, and feminine identity. Uncovering and acknowledging these agreements will help change the patterns that block your feminine vitality. When agreements become conscious, they can be renegotiated;

you can choose whether to continue with them or to change them. To help you recognize unconscious agreements that are limiting and in need of renegotiation, here are some examples:

### Personal Expression

I must hold back from my creative capacity because my parent/sibling/partner/friend/coworker/and so on, suppressed his or hers.

I have to hide my sadness or people will see how vulnerable I am.

I will suppress my vibrancy because it makes me feel out of control.

I will not be loved if I am angry.

I am not allowed to say what I feel.

I am not creative.

### Sense of Power

I will disconnect from my feminine power so that I do not threaten my parent/teacher/mentor/friend/and so on.

I am not able to create what I want.

Holding power is unsafe.

I cannot be both feminine and powerful.

My power comes from my connection to something, rather than from myself.

I am not allowed to express my true desires.

### Self-Worth

The world is not big enough for me to take up my share of space.

I am not allowed to be who I am.

I don't deserve to manifest my dreams.

I must take care of everyone's needs before I take care of myself.

I need to take what I can get because I am not worthy of
   receiving what I truly want.
I am valuable only when someone is attracted to me.

**Feminine Identity**
As a woman, I am not enough.
Femininity is a source of weakness.
My female body is a source of shame.
I will never be able to support myself financially.
It is not safe to express my feminine sensuality.
I cannot have both children and a career.
I am not allowed to be a leader.

Not only do unconscious agreements perpetuate long-term
patterns, they also prevent you from accessing your full feminine
potential. The internal conflict between the expansive nature of
your spirit and the restrictive nature of these agreements causes
tension in your body. This leads to imbalances in your energetic
and emotional realms. Boundaries created under the influence of
these agreements are self-limiting; such boundaries have been
formed in reaction to unhealthy beliefs and a restricted range,
rather than by the presence of a feminine radiance.

Identify the unconscious agreements in your life and begin
to make conscious transitions away from those that no longer
serve your well-being, moving toward those that honor and celebrate your feminine form.

### Exercise: Identifying Unconscious Agreements

1. Reflection: Select a topic such as creative expression, power,
   sensuality, self-worth, identity, or some other aspect of the
   feminine. Write continuously for ten minutes about your
   beliefs regarding this topic. Do not edit yourself, but write
   whatever comes to mind.

2. Ritual: Review your writing. Make a list of the agreements that are restricting your feminine nature. Rewrite these agreements into conscious statements that you want to live by. For example: take the belief *I have to dim my radiance to be safe* and transform it to *I proudly share my radiance with others.* Place these affirmations on an altar or in another designated space as a commitment to transformation.

## Receive Your Full Inheritance

By working with the lines that define your deepest patterns, you receive your full inheritance. The energy of your ancestors stands behind you as your strength, so you may call upon the ancestors to know your lineage and to support the creative energy in your body and your everyday life.

What is lineage when you carry the blood of people from a multitude of countries? What is lineage in a land of immigrants and their descendants, whose origins are distant or forgotten? What if you carry the blood of people who were enemies or who tried desperately to erase their ties to lineage? What about violence or shameful acts in your lineage?

Typically, I find that my clients accept parts of their lineage and disconnect—by blocking this energy in their bodies—from the rest. Afraid of passing on dysfunctional family patterns, women avoid these parts of their range. But reacting to lineage patterns by closing off from the pain of the past still ties a woman to her lineage, and as she resists the lineage energy in her body, it ceases to flow. The energy stagnates, and the woman is unable to transform its impact on her core. She may inadvertently continue the limiting pattern, in effect restricting her roles, self-definition, and potential, even causing her to live outside of her center.

Women worry about passing patterns on to their children or carrying these patterns themselves, yet this is the inevitable process of lineage. These imprints are purposeful, teaching us about the work of our family lines. Each person carries essential abilities and traits from her lineage. A child may look like a grandparent or an aunt or behave in a way that calls to mind a cousin. Lineage energy is meant to flow, allowing each generation access to its inheritance. Our best hope, for ourselves and our descendants, is to receive our full lineage energy and to build the structures to change and channel its flow.

### Women's Stories: Transforming a Lineage Pattern

Lucy came for pelvic work to support her overall health and reduce the tension patterns caused by uterine and ovarian cysts. I have noticed that cysts tend to occur in places of pelvic congestion, so increasing the cellular vitality in the pelvic bowl may assist a woman's healing. As I began to work on her pelvic alignment, I sensed the diminished presence in her core energy. It was as if she was sitting in front of her bowl rather than directly in her center. As I guided her awareness to the center of her body, Lucy realized that she did not pay much attention to this part of herself, particularly because she was not planning to have any children.

I explained the importance of her creative uterine and ovarian energies in various aspects of her life: forming dynamic relationships, establishing a fulfilling career, balancing the energy of work and home, making room for her creative pursuits, and maintaining her body's health and well-being. As she focused on her center, she also realized that she avoided this part of herself because it seemed associated with previous models of femininity that valued women primarily for caretaking roles or birthing children, which did not align with Lucy's image of herself.

I encouraged Lucy to maintain her presence in the center and establish a new creative pattern. By consciously reclaiming

her creative energies, she would create dynamic models of femininity and ways of being that would benefit future generations. We are best able to change lineage patterns and forge alternative paths by working with our bodies, where these patterns are held, to create the forms for the future.

## Reclaim Your Lineage

No matter what you know, seek your lineage. Reach beyond its living members. Listen until the voices of your ancestors are clear. Do not be afraid of the limiting aspects of your lineage; these regions are often awaiting reclamation. If there is discord with a family member or one of your lines, instead of focusing on the discord itself, do a ritual to grieve what was disrupted or lost. No matter how toxic the energy from a past event or pattern, there is full potential for healing—particularly when you invite the greater realm of spirit to reconnect with the place in the body where the energy is held. Call on the external support through friends, prayer, ritual, the elements of the earth; strengthen the flow of energy related to this line in your body. Smooth the overall energy current and it will restore, rather than disrupt, the energy in your life.

Do this all by working with the energy patterns in your body. Be compassionate with yourself and the patterns in your core that remind you of family patterns of dysfunction. The places where lineage patterns are broken or damaged, where the energy flows unsustainably, also contain untapped resources. The truth is that we cannot discount any part of our lineage, since rejecting a piece of lineage only results in profound self-denial. It is better to seek the aspects of our lineage that seem distasteful and begin to honor this forgotten ground. Bring back what was lost and, in doing so, repair your capacity to honor yourself and express your radiance. All your relationships and your creative energy will flow more easily when you receive the strength of your lineage lines. Reflections on reclaiming your lineage include:

What are the visible gifts of your lineage?

Where are there hidden gifts or sources of strength?

How does your body reflect the flow of your lineage energy?

How will you express or transform your inheritance?

*Women's Stories: Stepping into Her Mother Line*

Brianna came to see me when she was three months postpartum after birthing her first child. Her pelvic floor was weak, and she was unable to take care of her new baby without feeling the strain in her core. In my evaluation of her pelvic muscles, I noticed that she had little energetic presence in her root, particularly on the left, and that the left region of her pelvic muscles was hardly engaged. Her pelvis was slightly rotated, and I had the impression of her trying to avoid stepping into her left side. From the pattern in Brianna's body, I could read the energy strain along her mother line.

When a woman has her first child, it often brings her lineage work to the forefront, making the tension points in the lineage lines all the more obvious. Whether or not a woman has a child, however, her creative flow is enhanced by clearing the lineage strains held within her body. I asked Brianna how she was doing, and she told me that everything was fine, except that her mother was coming to visit. She and her mother had had a difficult relationship while Brianna was growing up, and Brianna knew that she wanted to mother her own child in a different way. The left side of Brianna's pelvis became more tense as she was talking, conveying the stress in her core.

I explained to Brianna that her best hope for changing a mothering pattern was to step fully into her left side and accept the lineage she had inherited. She was holding back on her left, the side of her mother, in an attempt to avoid the mistakes of the past. But with this much tension in her core, she would be less able to access the nurturance and inspiration from the receptive nature of the left side that was necessary to change the energetic form of a mothering pattern.

Learning about the tension in her root and wanting to address the dysfunction in her past, Brianna worked with the hesitation on the left side of her body. She imagined herself stepping boldly onto her left leg and encountered a rush of energy, a whole range of possibilities for her mothering. The tension in her left pelvic bowl released, and the muscles became more supple and responsive. I encouraged her to focus on what she needed from her mother line and then to ask for these needs to be met (either by someone directly or by spirit). We finished the pelvic care session with balance restored in her core. Brianna's pelvic muscles were fully engaged: instead of carrying the strain of the past, she could actively build for the future.

## Receive the Blessing of Your Ancestors

When reflecting upon your family, notice where you resist or hold back the ancestral energy in your core. You have greater resources to change the patterns of the past if you consciously receive and work with the energy of your lineage. The spirit of your lineage runs like a deep current in your body and will always bring fresh inspiration when you draw from its hidden lines and encourage this core energy to flow.

Remember your ancestors, once young and full of dreams. This is the energy that feeds your root. You are the hope of your lineage, the legacy of their creation. You are their prayer for the future, just as the next generation is your prayer. I invite you to call upon your ancestors with the following ritual blessing.

## Exercise: Ancestor Blessing

1. Reflection: Take a moment to ponder the ancestors who stand behind you as a part of your lineage tree. Gather photos and place them on an altar, speak your ancestors' names, or simply sense their energy behind you.

2. Ritual: Light three candles—one for the past, one for the present, and one for the future. Speak the following Ancestor Blessing:

> *I call on the women and men of my mother line.*
> *I call on the women and men of my father line.*
> *I call on the lineages of those who have supported my journey in this life.*
> *I call on the spirits of this land.*
> *Bring your strength, your beauty, your dreams, your joy to me—the one who now carries on the work of our lineage.*
> *Bring energy and light to my life so that I may do this work of transforming wounds, nurturing hope, celebrating joy, and sharing love;*
> *I am building the structures and sowing the seeds of a bountiful life for myself and for all who will come after me.*
> *Know that your life and energy, all of your steps, were a blessing.*
> *May you rest in peace, held by spirit.*
> *The light that you carried lives on.*
> *I honor you, ancestors.*

*I give thanks for you.*
*I ask for your blessing, your energy, to flow—*
*like a sacred river—through my body and*
*life.*

Integrate the energy of your lineage into your life. Carefully sort through what you have been given so you may reinvent the possibilities for yourself and your future creations. You expand your creative range when you know how to interact with this history upon which you stand.

*May you receive the blessing of your life.*

# SEVEN

# Discovering Your Full Feminine Range

*In the past, a woman had to choose whether to use her creative energy in the home or the workplace. Though we have more choices now, many women are still running these divisive energy patterns. Instead, a woman's creative energy is designed to flow through all areas of her life: to inspire, to heal, to expand her creative potential. This chapter shares the concept of each woman making her own root medicine to restore the full capacity of her creative life. Women no longer need to choose between home and work— in fact, both women and men (and children) need more dynamic forms to serve the vast nature of who they truly are.*

*T*hese things I love: the wooden spatula in my hand bumping against the cast-iron skillet, the milky warmth of hot coffee and cream, the deep hues of my sons' eyes, bare feet padding across the floor, the crunch of dark chocolate, the smell of red wine pouring into a glass, the weight of a wool blanket covering my baby and me, his dream-filled breath against my chest while I turn the crisp pages of a new book.

When I indulge my senses in these and other ways, my female body responds. My womb is warm, my center relaxed, my root soft and supple. I inhabit the still point within a moment, or by following a quickened pace from within; I delightfully engage my extra creative capacity to accomplish tasks with lightning speed.

However, when I push myself to race against the clock or willfully trudge through chore after chore, my body tightens in rebellion. The state of my wild self is a direct measure of my present relationship with desire.

It has taken several years for me to reinhabit my own desires and to even understand desire as a way to meet with spirit through my body. It required dismantling expectations from society and various people whom I had wanted to please, whose agendas I mistakenly took to be my own. Piece by piece, I replaced the goals of others and outer measures of success with my own sense of purpose and intention. Where I previously took direction from external sources, I now turn my attention inward, to my own root, for the guidance that I seek. I have learned my body's instinctive response to a natural creative flow. I am more content now, satisfying my real needs for expressive creativity and tangible sensuality that bring me into direct contact with spirit.

When I think of untamed wildness, my two-year-old son comes to mind. He embodies desire in its purest form. He wants to pour water and feel it moving over his fingers. He climbs into my lap, touching, scooping, and tasting the food on my plate. One morning I found him standing, barefoot, on a banana. With a wide grin on his face, he repeated, "Squish, squish," as the white of the banana spread between his toes. Every drawer, every object, is the subject of his exploration. Like most two-year-olds, he wants to be touched and held, to hear stories or songs; his desire is an insatiable hunger.

In modern culture, desire often goes unmet. Not for lack; we have an abundance of goods designed to fill every appetite. But to appease our true appetite, we must pause, taking a moment to fill our senses with what they crave: the aroma of food, the gaze of a loved one, a touch of skin or earth. We must pause and be fed to be able to receive the abundance all around us. To be fed, we must know what we are hungry for.

## Reclaim Your Desire

At the root of every desire is a longing for union. We feed our bodies' desire to remember a sense of connection, for we long to reexperience the oneness we knew in our mother's womb. There, we were fed, we were part of another. Our hunger for sustenance begins in any separation we felt in the womb and, significantly, when we are born. Satisfying our desire is an attempt to feed this hunger; it is our way of reaching for something which will sustain us.

Desire often becomes confused with sexuality, portrayed as dangerous, dirty, and shameful. But desire is related to the sensual nature of the body. In its authentic state, desire is the physical expression of what is, at heart, a longing for spiritual connection—the link between spirit and form.

### Women's Stories: Restoring Her Sense of Desire

Shana came to see me with a long history of pelvic issues and an inability to have pleasurable sex. She wanted to work on her body to increase her connection with her partner, but first we had to discover what her body was trying to convey.

Looking at her family history for patterns, Shana told me that her mother and two sisters did not have any pelvic concerns. But she said they also seemed to be more disconnected from their bodies. She was the one in her family most likely to be honest about difficult situations and was known for her tendency to "tell it like it is." Shana also mentioned that her mother had been sexually abused as a child by both of her parents, and Shana felt that some of her own body issues and sexual inhibition were related to this past abuse.

I asked her to bring her attention to her root. As Shana began to focus on her pelvis, she felt disoriented, so I encouraged her to guide her awareness back to her body. As she did so, she noticed that it was hard for her to take a breath. I encouraged her to breathe as fully as possible and to pay attention to her body as we worked on her pelvic bowl.

The energy that was moving as Shana connected with her body felt sticky and overwhelming to her, which is typical when there is a family history of sexual abuse. Even though Shana was not abused herself, the energy of her mother's experience of abuse may have registered in her body. For Shana's mother, her childhood joy had been overwhelmed by the sexual abuse from her parents. Adult sexuality contains a heaviness that a child's energy system is not equipped to deal with. Shana's mother likely carried this heaviness in her body, and Shana's own body registered an energy imprint of the same pattern. Children's bodies often reflect the energy patterns of their parents because initially they have no boundaries; they do not differentiate themselves from either parent—but especially from their mother if they were held in her womb.

As an adult, Shana could clear the family abuse energy from her body. Containing the abuse energy from her maternal line drained Shana's energy and dampened her sense of desire. Rather than inhabiting her own energy potential, Shana's pelvic energy system was constantly guarding against the imprint of toxic abuse energy. I directed her to her uterus, a powerful organ for releasing burdensome energies. In the next several sessions, Shana cleared her body by breathing into her uterus and using her uterine capacity for releasing energy. We also worked with Shana's ovarian energy to increase her pelvic boundaries and identify what core energy was hers and what belonged to others.

As Shana clarified the energy of her pelvic bowl, she recovered her own wants and needs. She desired more color on her walls and regular massage sessions for her body. Rather than the heaviness she was accustomed to in her center, she now felt lighter and more alive. She began to explore her tastes and senses. This exploration translated into a deeper intimacy with her partner. For the first time, she began to find her own desire for sex. Shana realized that in all her previous encounters with this and other partners, sex was initiated and shaped by the desire of another. Just as with her body connection, she was letting others define her experience without regard for herself. By paying attention to her body, Shana followed her own desire for connection. And as she found her cravings in other areas, she discovered her appetite for sexuality as well.

## Unhealthy Forms of Desire

In the absence of a true connection to spirit or the feminine within us, many unhealthy forms of desire arise from the damage and distortion to our authentic nature. Taking place over several generations, these distortions often give rise to addictions. Addictions and other incessant cravings signal that we are living with profound disruptions or severe imbalances in the energy field where vital energy is dissipated. Women, and men, can be addicted to praise, attention, food, sex, material goods, gambling, power, rage, work, and so on, but they are responding to a hunger that occurs because their energy is draining away.

Though it is the energy field, and the relationship with spirit, that is in need of repair, most people attempt to either fill the hunger by feeding their addiction or block it by resisting the unhealthy desire. If you discover a desire that, when fed, only results in a bigger appetite or greater feelings of emptiness, then your energy field and your feminine nature need care. Instead of filling a void, remember the deeper flow that—when restored—will sustain you. The only way to truly achieve freedom from these unhealthy forms of desire, and other toxic patterns, is to attend to the energy disruptions and imbalances (and grieve the losses) that create them. In doing so, you often heal essential patterns in your body and your lineage energy flow.

## Clarifying Sexual Desire

Sexual desire should have a very specific place. It belongs between two consenting adults who ideally understand the power of their union and its potential to create new life. This fusion of male and female (regardless of actual gender) is holy. Like all holy things, it should be reserved for clear, conscious, and intentional use.

Great pain is caused by misplaced or misused sexual desire. When it is used for power over another person, it is detrimental for all involved. If you have been the victim of unwanted sexual desires or have coupled with disrespectful partners, clear out your energy system. If you are longing for a partner to fill a void, redirect your focus back to your own center. Take courage and gather the resources—personal rituals; friends; counselors; bodyworkers; energy healers; body-based practices like yoga, Pilates, or tai chi; and so on—to assist you in restoring a healthy connection to your body. You will inevitably encounter your authentic desire (which refuels your body with fresh chi and a connection to the deeper energy currents of the spiritual realm) and rediscover a source of profound nourishment and joy.

The basis of a healthy sexuality—and positive associations with other intimate bodily experiences like eating, menstruating, birthing, and breastfeeding—is a healthy relationship with sensuality (your ability to receive sensory information through the body). Learn to recognize the difference between sensuality and sexuality, and how they relate to one another in your life. Notice where you restrict your sensuality, or ability to experience pleasure, because of fears about sexuality. Likewise, wherever your sexuality is blocked, restore your sensual expression and observe what changes. By actively paying attention to your senses, you can increase your overall sensory awareness and enhance your bodily delight with any experience.

## Exercise: Opening Your Senses

1. Take a moment and pay attention to your body. Whether you are in a quiet space or in the midst of a busy home or office, stop for a moment, close your eyes, and feel the overall state of your body. Let your thoughts pass by like clouds, and dip into the sensory realm of your body.

2. Notice how your breath travels and where it flows naturally. Bring your breath to any areas in your body that feel tight. Spend a few minutes noticing and expanding your breath.

3. Pay attention to your sensation of touch. Notice the texture of clothing on your skin. Feel where you are sitting or how your body is meeting the ground. Is your body warm or cold? Is your body touching something hard or soft?

4. Take a deep breath through your nose and notice if you smell anything. Is the air fresh? Is it warm or cold?

5. Listen for sounds. What do you notice? Are there noises that you have been hearing but not noticing, tuning them out in some way?

6. Open your eyes and find something to take in with your vision. Look at a bright picture or the scenery outside; observe the colors of your food or the patterns in a room.

7. Extend this exercise by preparing a meal, talking with a friend, making love, or going for a walk with your senses on alert, and notice how your experience deepens and your body responds.

Explore your sensual desire for connection by more consciously taking nourishment through food, relationships, and the inspirations of spirit. Sexual desire arises from sensuality, but sensuality is not always sexual. Eating is sensual. Touch is sensual. Too often we rush through the experiences of our bodies without really sensing (feeling with our senses) the various textures of the experience. Depriving or denying our sensual nature is in fact detrimental to our sexuality, our relationships, the health of our bodies, and our ability to determine our own needs and desires.

Awareness of your bodily senses is essential to be able to nourish yourself and feed your desire. Nourishment requires that you have a healthy relationship with your hunger and your deepest longings as a woman. If you have learned to feed others instead of yourself, and if this has happened for generations of women in your line, the hunger can be overwhelming when you first turn to face it. But if you learn what it is that your body and being craves and how to provide this for yourself, you will experience a dynamic flow with your creative essence and root desire. Further reflections regarding desire include:

What are your deepest desires as a woman?
Where is your desire met and where are you still yearning?
How do you like to indulge your senses?
How do you express or restrict your sensuality?
How does your relationship with sensuality affect your sexuality, your creative flow, your connection to spirit, and other bodily experiences?

## Rage: Voice Your Needs

As women begin to listen to their vaginas and pelvic spaces, I often hear them express surprise at the amount of anger they find. Anger, to the point of rage, is one of the most common emotions held in the pelvic space. A woman's root will rage in response to betrayals, experiences of power loss, and the unmet needs that diminish her wild feminine spirit.

Exploring her root, a woman may discover pelvic anger in reaction to being female. Rage may arise when a woman's sense of her own power does not match the opportunities for women presented by her family or culture. Feelings of bodily betrayal when experiencing pelvic pain, menstrual pain, or infertility are also common sources of internal rage. Wherever a woman encounters her rage, she also finds the potential to address her needs and to fulfill her desires.

## The Root Voice of Rage: Unheard Cries

The first encounter with your own root voice of rage may be startling in its intensity. After hearing it a few times, though, you may notice the clarity with which this voice alerts you to any need, potential boundary violation, or tendency to give away your power. A valuable ally to help you guard your space, this root voice is worth listening to.

When regularly acknowledged, your root anger will be expressed calmly: *No taking on that project right now—your plate is presently full.* However, if frequently ignored, your root voice may increase her volume: *How could you do this when you know how exhausted you are?* Or she may collapse and leave you internally frustrated and undefended: *Fine, you are not listening to me so I'm leaving—but do not blame me for the consequences.* Begin to notice the presence of anger in your own root voice. Reflections to help you do this include:

When do you hear your root voice of rage?
What is your root presently raging about?
Do you listen to her wise words?

## Why All These Raging Vaginas?

The vagina and pelvic space hold essential feminine wisdom for every woman. However, when there are places of disconnection between a woman and her root voice, this resource remains untapped. Like an unacknowledged friend, the mouthiest part of the root, the vagina, feels unappreciated and rageful—particularly when she observes a woman selling herself short.

Whenever a woman chooses to forgo her root wisdom and deny the full range of her needs, she is giving away her power. A woman may choose to do this in exchange for something she believes necessary. For example, previous generations of women lost some of their power because they were dependent upon receiving financial security from their husbands. Though basic material needs were provided for and they received a sense of security, many women suppressed their strong voices and creative potentials. When women deny themselves in order to fulfill real or imagined needs, they spend most of their time outside of their true creative range. The descendants of these women are left to find their way back to the root, to what holds meaning for them, and must sort through these core patterns.

Prolonged self-denial acts like a pressure cooker, creating a toxic buildup of internal rage. This often overlies a well of grief, and if unmourned, it simmers, at times boiling over and burning all those in close proximity. The daughters of women who have denied themselves in some way will experience the full intensity of this rage in themselves as they explore, and begin to recover, lost ground. As they renegotiate issues of power loss, challenge myths about financial dependence, or reconnect to the pelvic space, they will encounter all the previously unmet needs of their female lineage.

Whenever a woman changes inherited physical, emotional, or mental patterns of womanhood, she must face the unheard cries of her ancestors. She must be strong in order to retrieve the latent gifts of her lineage. Listening to the root voice will guide a woman to the personal or generational power-related issues that need to be addressed before she can reclaim her own feminine range.

### Women's Stories: Finding Her Place of Power

Caitlyn came to improve her pelvic strength. In her assessment, I found that, indeed, her root muscles were weak. There was only a hint of movement when she tightened her muscles and little pelvic presence or energetic vitality. This was a pelvic pattern of energetic collapse, indicating difficulty accessing personal power or self-advocating.

During our session, Caitlyn mentioned that she was frustrated at work because she felt invalidated. As she spoke, her pelvic tension increased noticeably. After bringing this to her attention, I asked Caitlyn to envision a situation in which she felt empowered. She called to mind her practice of yoga, and her pelvic tension released while her pelvic presence, including changes in the warmth and suppleness of her muscles, improved significantly. She was accessing her pelvic power. Caitlyn continued to practice feeling the difference between her pelvic tension and pelvic power.

At the end of the session, she was able to tighten her pelvic muscles across a greater range. As we finished, she told me she wanted to teach yoga full-time but had stayed in her current job for financial security. She now realized the physical and energetic consequences of compromising herself and leaving her own desires unmet, and that continuing to access the power in her root would encourage her to operate from a place of power in her life.

By attending to her center, a woman will be clear about her desires and more likely to find the opportunities that truly sustain her. When a woman feels a power deficit in her life, it is often because she is out of touch with her creative essence. Lack of power may seem like a normal state if that is all she has known, or she may be focused on external situations in her life, making her unaware of how to align herself with the power to direct her creative capacity. I encouraged Caitlin to turn inward and to remember the powerful energy that flows from her center and gives form to her life.

## More Angry Vaginas: Raging against Boundary Violations

Boundary violations are personal invasions, and they are frequently registered by the vagina and pelvic space. When safety is compromised and trust is broken, outrage is a healthy response. If parents or other adults did not protect, or perhaps violated, a woman's boundaries as a child, she may subconsciously allow others to continue these violations. The vagina will rage, however, and try to restore the protective response the woman herself was unable to make at that time.

Any pelvic experience that a woman does not fully agree to is a potential boundary violation. Such violations can include sexual encounters, all forms of abuse, medical procedures, abortions, or other situations in which a woman was unable to fully access her personal power. It is important to acknowledge and heal these traumatic events, both for a woman's vital self and for any future partners or children. Otherwise, these events disrupt the energy of her pelvic bowl, limiting her connection with her body and with others.

*Women's Stories: Acknowledging Her Root Voice*

When Lisa came to my office, she was two months postpartum and experiencing painful sexual intercourse. She had a fairly common history: a mild tear during childbirth was repaired with stitches and was now further irritated by pelvic penetration. Her root was speaking to her, but she did not hear what it was saying.

Six weeks after the birth of her child, at her postpartum pelvic exam, Lisa had agreed to a recommendation from her primary care provider to address the pain of intercourse. This procedure involved cutting the scar tissue forming near the stitches in her vaginal wall. Lisa described the procedure as "more painful than childbirth," and it only seemed to worsen her pelvic pain. Now, as I began the pelvic release and vaginal massage to encourage her body's healing process, I asked Lisa to listen to the internal messages from her body. Lisa said that her vagina was "pissed." In bringing her awareness to it, she felt that she owed her body an apology because she never consulted her own intuition before making this health-care decision.

I used vaginal massage and taught Lisa self-massage techniques. We were able to restore pelvic balance and relieve her postpartum pain. Additionally, since Lisa was now listening to her body, she was able to receive the messages it held for her. Had she not learned to hear the voice of her root, her body rage might eventually have been released unconsciously, toward her partner or herself. By listening to her root, she brought the knowledge of its anger to a conscious—and therefore transformable—level. Consciousness brings clarity, healing, and the potential for transformation.

## Addressing and Alleviating Pelvic Pain

As more women listen to their roots, they will learn how pelvic care can gently and respectfully address pain and other pelvic symptoms. I find that skilled application of vaginal massage alleviates various types of pain. One of my clients was in her fifties and had lived with painful intercourse for over twenty years. On her fourth appointment with me, she came to my office with tears in her eyes, reporting that she had experienced her first pain-free sex ever, after just three treatment sessions of vaginal massage. My eyes teared as well, both in celebration of her landmark and with a sense of sadness that something so simple might have alleviated her pain years prior.

It is always important to have pelvic pain evaluated by a primary care physician to rule out any overall health concerns, but many times it is caused by pelvic imbalances and chronic tension patterns that can be addressed by a skilled practitioner. Pelvic pain can arise from past injuries and traumas or as an emotional form of armoring in response to early experiences of abuse. I have seen women have pelvic pain as a form of unconscious protection when their partner was disrespectful or unfaithful, that later resolved when they ended the relationship or discovered the truth. Or when a woman stays in a marriage or relationship where she is unfulfilled or unable to express herself, there can also be pelvic pain. Additionally, pain such as twinges in the ovaries or tender places in the muscles can arise as a woman begins to change her core patterns and strengthen her organ energy flow while the body adjusts to a new way of being.

I continue to see many women who have painful intercourse after childbirth because of a tear that required stitches and the resulting scar tissue. These women are routinely told that their symptoms are normal and may resolve with time. Instead they suffer or stop having sex altogether, and then find their way to my office through a referral. When their pain is resolved after a few sessions of bodywork, we wonder together why the root of the body continues to receive less care than it deserves.

I have assisted many women in alleviating pelvic pain by working with pelvic tension patterns and trigger points, educating them about the contributing factors to pelvic pain, encouraging them to create relationships that are honoring and supportive of their full expression, and teaching them how to listen and align themselves with their own root voice.

## Hear Your Root Voice of Rage

Boundary violations and power losses occur when the root of the female body remains unheard. When you express your root voice of rage with others, you may encounter responses like, "What's the big deal?" "Why are you making such an issue about it?" "Let it go," and so on. These statements encourage you to suppress your strong voice of rage. However, suppressing this voice makes it impossible for you to advocate for yourself. Your energy is spent holding back your expression instead of responding to the warnings from your root voice. Reflections to help you hear your root voice of rage include:

> What does your root say?
> What happened when you did not listen?
> Have you ever been criticized when you were expressing the needs of your female body or feminine self?
> What other forms of expression have been suppressed that you want to access again?

## Let Your Root Talk

The antidote to suppression is expression. To begin restoring the expressive voice of your root, look to your emotional holding patterns. These can include issues that you tend to avoid, people who put you on guard, or particular feelings you hide. Notice where in your life there is a flow of open communication and where your ability to communicate is blocked. Notice especially how these patterns relate to issues impacting your feminine identity, boundaries, or self-expression. By paying attention to your bodily and feminine needs, particularly those that have gone unfulfilled, your root finds its voice. When you listen to the core of your body and your root voice, you open a whole new range of feminine expression in your life. Reflections on letting your root talk include:

When has your root voice been suppressed?
How does it continue to be unheard or repressed?
What is needed to restore your root voice?

As you begin to listen to your root voice, you will be able to release old rage and clarify your true needs. You will be more readily alerted to toxic situations, boundary violations, and other issues that would otherwise drain your personal power—and you'll be able to rectify them. In doing so, you discover your true power—the power to be fully yourself, engaged in the life you desire.

### Exercise: Identifying Power Loss

To reclaim your ability to advocate for yourself, it is essential to revisit the times when your power was taken or given up.

1. Reflection: Make a list of instances in which you were violated, unheard, or in any way stripped of your personal power. Next to the event, write the specific words that identify what was lost (voice, integrity, safety, joy, value, and so on). Also note whether or not your power was restored in some way at a later time. Acknowledge what it was that helped you reclaim your power.

2. Ritual: On the other side of your paper, describe what you would like to reclaim from the particular aspect of power that was lost, and place it on an altar or visible space. For example: If your voice was lost, vow to speak up in the next situation that takes courage. Be compassionate with the parts of yourself that were wounded. Find an activity or gesture to continue the process of reclaiming the power of your words, body, spirit, or other aspects of your feminine self.

## Renegotiate Your Relationships

When you utilize your creative energy, you are naturally drawn to others in intimate, personal, and even professional relationships. In order to reclaim your creative energy, examine these partnerships. There is an energy exchange—a giving and receiving—that takes place in a vibrant relationship, but when a relationship only takes energy and gives little in return, this may diminish your vitality. When you listen for the root voice of rage, you can identify the situations or expectations that maintain unsustainable patterns and begin to renegotiate how you relate to others.

The process of renegotiating your relationships may require taking apart old structures or challenging family communication patterns to tell the stories or ask the questions that need to be heard. Be prepared for any action you take to cause a reaction; when you change the way you relate to others, they also change. Starting the process with trusted women friends or a counselor may make renegotiating your relationships a little easier. In our shared courage to break unhealthy ties, we find the freedom we desire. No one is truly free unless we are all liberated from the destructive habits that threaten the wild feminine. You may find that some unhealthy relationships fall away as you do your work in this area.

I have also seen that the most real and lasting changes in a woman's creative relationships will arise by primarily working on her root patterns. When a woman redefines her root patterns, she influences the way others are drawn to her and how those currently in her life interact with her. Rather than engaging in conflict or other direct exchange, she shifts the underlying energy patterns, and all her relationships shift as well.

For example, several of my clients have expressed sexual frustration and their desire for a strong male partner. Or they want to be attended to and recognized in some way. They ask for more attention from their partner, but it is unsuccessfully received as criticism and results in no visible change in the relationship. However, when one of these same women works on receiving more of her feminine energy and plays with her feminine expression, she has direct access to the responsive energy she craves. Suddenly, her partner is also noticing her radiance. The nature of their relationship changes because instead of a sense of scarcity that leaves a woman pulling and prodding her partner, there is now an abundance of creative energy between them—and the energy itself has more charge, clarity, and potential. Likewise, if a woman has a difficult relationship with one of her family members, working with the tension in her core that relates to her sense of power, self-expression, security, access to joy, or some other aspect (that also seems to correlate to her relationship) will reduce tension in the relationship as well.

When a woman does not receive what she wants in a given relationship, she often holds those closest to her accountable with tension in her core. This continues to limit her ability to make or receive what she wants for herself. It is better to release the tension in her core, releasing her expectations as well. Then the true energy movement begins. There is less tension in her relationships, allowing more energy and, ultimately, love to flow. Rather than trying to fix someone or waiting for them to change in order to acknowledge a woman's capabilities or fulfill her desires, she finds access to the energy or resources within her own body. The ones whom she has released respond to the freedom and flow of energy as well, and she may be surprised at the unexpected transformations and joyful reconnections that arise.

## Women's Stories: Sifting through the Ashes of Rage

Leslie came to my clinic to address pelvic tension, and as she connected to her pelvic space, she found rage. She found seemingly limitless rage. Over the next several months, every time she listened to her root, it ranted and railed. It protested when she consented to sex she did not truly want. It complained when she had a deadline and worked overtime. It exploded when someone—anyone—asked her for something she did not have the energy to give.

When she realized the amount of pent-up frustration and anger she had not been acknowledging, Leslie thought it no wonder that her muscles were tense. As she began to listen, her pelvic muscles relaxed and over time her root voice softened. Beneath the ashes of her rage, she discovered a tendency toward self-denial and a profound sadness for the self-sacrifices she had made in the process of developing a career.

Leslie's root voice was leading her back to her vital essence, and she followed it. She recognized how much her work had taken over her life. She wanted to be successful and took on responsibility for far more than she could do, thus compromising her own needs. Her self-care and her family bore the brunt of this self-denial, and she gave all her best energy to the workplace.

As Leslie began to put limits on her work commitments, she had more space for the rest of her life. Her rage disappeared. Leslie's anger had been a signal of her extreme depletion; pushing others away out of exhaustion rather than taking charge of her own energy from the beginning. Now she began to take time for her own needs and desires. She enjoyed cooking and began coming home early from work to make dinner. She started taking a dance class and set up time to walk regularly with a friend. With all these changes, Leslie found that her pelvic muscles were significantly less tense. In addressing her pelvic needs, she also recovered her core desire to enjoy life outside of the workplace.

## Move into Righteous Rage

Righteous rage, as author and storyteller Clarissa Pinkola Estes describes in *Women Who Run with the Wolves*, is the fuel that propels a woman forward through the collective silence and fear to reclaim and protect her rightful place. Righteous rage is a catalyst for breaking down old forms or ways of living that no longer serve a purpose, and it assists with the creation of new forms.

Righteous rage helps a woman take up space in the world and find her own unique contribution. It alerts her to patterns of the past that must be changed before she can embody her full potential. It is the will to cultivate relationships that fulfill and nourish her feminine spirit. This type of rage is healthy—it tells others to make room because she intends to protect her boundaries.

Rage arises when a woman is not heard, seen, touched, supported, and honored in the ways she wants and needs, as woman, mother, daughter, sister, lover, and partner. Sometimes you have to keep digging to find the righteous rage that will help you say what you mean and ask for what you need. Dig deep, until you find the soulful voice that can be heard when you listen to your root place.

Righteous rage can be channeled into the building of new structures that support your growth, fulfill your desires, and help to create a vibrant and deeply satisfying life. Reflections on rage include:

Where and how do you advocate for yourself?
Where do you want to get louder in your life?
What need or desire is your righteous rage guiding you toward?

## Vaginal Energy and Your Wild Feminine

By reconnecting to the physical root of her body, a woman recovers the essential aspects of her feminine nature. In these reconnections, reunions of body and spirit, we first glimpse the wild feminine. While the vagina is primarily considered a sexual place, it is much more. The vagina is the doorway of life, a connection to the fierce essence that is woman. It guards the space where a woman gestates her seeds, and this guarding ensures that there is abundant energy for a woman's own creative inspirations. Sensuality, creativity, and ultimately joy arise naturally when a woman is present and engaged in her vaginal energy, her own wild feminine.

Containing the cycle of regeneration, the energy of the vagina is either open to receive or closed and guarding what is precious to a woman. This is the place in the female body that responds to a woman's primitive or natural instincts. When she is able to access the full range of her vaginal energy, she gains a powerful tool for replenishing her feminine radiance and protecting her feminine self.

Listening to the response of the vagina that tightens when it does not feel safe, you will hear the voice of your guardian: *Don't even think about taking in that toxic energy.* Likewise, you may also cultivate the receptive powers of your vagina when you hear, *Ah, now that's refreshing; to bring a specific energy into your life.*

**Vaginal Energy: Open to Receive**
Receptivity is one of the true gifts of femininity. It allows a woman to take in energy and transform it. This feminine quality is the basis for a woman's fertility, whether it is expressed through having children or by realizing her creative visions. When the vagina is open, indicating a more receptive root, a woman is more able to take energy into her body—whether as the sensual energy of the sun on her skin or the physical contact of a partner. Her vagina is also the passageway that opens in order for the womb to release menstrual blood, clear energy from the pelvic bowl, or birth a baby. Ponder the receptive nature of the vagina and the feminine with these questions:

What would you like to receive into your life?
Is there anything that you are blocking yourself from
    receiving?

What is needed for you to be more receptive or to receive
what you want?

The following exercise can be done to enhance the receptive
qualities of your root. Use it to help you receive the energy you
desire, prepare your body for conception, or simply soften your
core and increase your receptive powers.

### Exercise: Enhancing Your Receptivity

Read through the exercise first, and then close your eyes to begin.
Find a comfortable position, sitting or lying down.

1. Guide your attention internally to your pelvic space and
   observe any sensations that arise. Inhale and sense any places
   of holding or tension; exhale and release or soften these places.

2. Gradually, with each breath, soften the whole vagina, from
   the opening to the deepest parts. The energy of your body
   responds to your breath. Place your hand over your low
   belly, and focus your attention on any areas of tension that
   persist. Imagine walking around your bowl and inviting the
   energy to be soft like clouds.

3. Visualize what you would like to receive as a woman. Continue to soften the layers of your pelvic bowl. Inhale and
   draw in fresh energy to revitalize your root and enliven your
   creative vision; exhale and continue to release any resistance.
   With each cycle, let the beauty around you fill your whole
   energy field. Repeat five to seven times.

4. Give thanks for your root and for your potential to receive
   vibrant energy into your body and life. Open your eyes and
   notice any changes in your vagina and pelvic bowl.

## Vaginal Energy: Closed in Protection

Socialization generally encourages girls and women to be polite instead of responding to situations based on their intuition or body signals; this ultimately limits their ability to defend themselves. Body signals that warn of danger include a sudden heightening of awareness and tightening in the pelvic floor or throat musculature; these muscles react similarly when a woman is threatened. If a woman is unaware of these intuitive signals and their meaning, her safety is compromised physically or even energetically. Learn the signs of your protective vaginal energy in order to access your own core guardian. Teach children to honor the wisdom of a protective response in their bodies rather than to ignore their intuition, which can lead to compromising themselves.

The guardian nature of the vagina is a valuable asset. Too often, women give away their energy in order to please or satisfy others. Actions taken out of obligation carry an undercurrent of resentment, and tension builds in the root when a woman denies her own needs. It is better to listen to the guardian in your core. When you guard your body and your creative energy as precious, you will only give of yourself in an authentic and sustainable way. Use these questions to ponder the protective response of your vagina in guarding your feminine self:

When have you honored your protective instincts?
What have you been taking in that you would rather guard against?
When have you given something and compromised your own needs?
What is needed to activate your core guardian?

Enhance your ability to guard your space with the following exercise.

## Exercise: Activating Your Core Guardian

Read through the exercise first, and then close your eyes to begin. Find a comfortable position, sitting or lying down.

1. Guide your attention internally to your pelvic bowl and observe your sense of well-being. This is your inner sacred space and should be a place of comfort and security.

2. Visualize your pelvic bowl and notice whether any part feels too open or unprotected. If you find a region in need of your vaginal guarding energy, ask your root what source of protection will assist you. The most potent protection is your full presence—call your root energy back to fill your pelvic bowl. Visualize it passing though one of the elements, like fire or water, to revitalize and clear the energy as it returns.

3. What is the essence of your core guardian? For some women, their protective energy appears as a certain color or quality of energy. Others see a protective image or animal spirit. However your core guardian appears, invite these aspects of your fierce wild feminine to protect you. This is your space. Ask for any additional protection you feel is needed.

4. When you feel present and protected in your core, identify your own needs. When necessary, respond to a situation from this place in yourself where you feel confident and safe. Ask spirit to send a wave of healing light out to all beings. Less protection is required when everyone is whole.

5. Honor the wisdom of your guarding energy. Open your eyes and notice any changes in your vagina and pelvic bowl.

## Patterns of Vaginal Energetic Imbalance

A woman's feminine wounds are visible in her patterns of vaginal energetic imbalance, such as excess receptivity or heightened guarding. Any situation that has compromised a woman's sense of security, including previous physical, sexual, or emotional abuse, will cause vaginal or root imbalances, which can reveal where her access to her wild feminine is restricted. Paying attention to the guardian in her root will restore a woman to her rightful range.

## Excess Vaginal Receptivity

One pattern of energetic imbalance in the vagina is excess vaginal receptivity. After the birth of a baby, this receptive pattern is normal for three to four months as a woman continues to receive the energy for her baby and her mothering. Likewise, this pattern may occur to bring in new energy after the completion of any life transition or major creative cycle. Enhanced receptivity is also normal after a miscarriage, and in my own life felt like a sacred time—when I received many blessings and lessons into my life. But any prolonged period of excess vaginal receptivity will begin to overwhelm or drain a woman's core energy, because her body is continuously open, rather than following the more sustainable pattern that alternates between opening to receive and then closing to integrate new information and energy.

If a woman has a vaginal imbalance resulting from past trauma, she may unconsciously prolong the pattern by receiving energy indiscriminately, engaging in sex or other forms of energetic exchange without regard for her true needs. Because she is not protecting herself, the energy of her pelvis becomes cloudy and her life lacks clarity. She also has difficulty maintaining her energy or sustaining her creations. Physical symptoms of excess vaginal receptivity include a decreased ability to tighten or engage pelvic muscles and dampened vaginal sensation or areas of numbness in the pelvic muscles. Reflections regarding excess vaginal receptivity include:

Have you ever received energy into the root that you did
   not want?
How would you like to clear this energy and restore your
   guardian?
Have you ever experienced the enhanced receptivity available after birthing a baby or moving through an intensely
   creative period?
What energy moved into or cleared from your life with
   each birth experience or creative movement?

*Women's Stories: Accessing the Guardian Energy of the Vagina*

Sarah came for pelvic work after the birth of her child. Her
evaluation revealed weakened pelvic muscles and an overall
decrease in vaginal tone. She was exhausted and reported that
sex was not as pleasurable as it had been because she had a
"wide-open sensation" in her vagina.

   Childbirth can stretch the vaginal wall and change the
shape of the vagina (which vaginal massage can significantly
reduce). However, something else was prolonging this pattern
in Sarah's body, as we discovered while doing pelvic work.

   When Sarah began to engage her muscles, they were initially slow to respond. She had difficulty sensing the various
pelvic quadrants, and there was a diminished energetic presence
in her pelvic space. The lack of physical and energetic engagement in her core made for a poor container: her core energy
was leaking from her pelvic bowl, leaving her continuously
fatigued.

   I asked Sarah to visualize a few ways to give herself more
support during her daily mothering tasks. She imagined herself resting during her baby's naps and taking time to savor
some of the spontaneous moments with her baby, instead
of rushing to complete the household tasks, and her pelvic

muscles twitched in response. Her pelvic energy became noticeably stronger.

As Sarah pondered her mothering routine, she recognized an internal struggle. She wanted to enjoy her baby, but was accustomed to being highly productive and keeping her house in order. The constant care of her baby and extra needs from her postpartum body slowed her overall pace to a level she had never experienced. She struggled to reconcile her need to accomplish tangible goals with the fact that the caretaking that occupied her days was largely unmeasurable. Likewise, many of her extended family members had visited to meet the new baby, leaving Sarah and her partner to make meals and host many more people than they had energy for. When she focused on her pelvic bowl and felt her own depleted energy, she discovered that she was placing the needs of her visitors and the upkeep of her home before the well-being of herself and her baby. She was expending her energy based on prior expectations of herself rather than paying attention to the internal locus that would accurately assess her mothering capacity.

Sarah needed to guard her energy more carefully and acknowledge the load she was already carrying as she restored her body from the expenditures of pregnancy and birth and tended a new baby. I encouraged Sarah to visualize her pelvic bowl and imagine holding her baby there, centering on what was most essential during this sacred post-birth time when a woman is still open and receiving energy from spirit. As she did so, her pelvic muscles began to pulse. She was activating her "mama bear" energy, the instinctive response in the root that protects a new mom and baby (or any woman doing her deep and private creative work). At the end of our session, Sarah had more sensation and engagement in the muscles of her root and a better container to hold her vital energy.

Over the next few weeks, she could feel the difference in her root strength whenever she cherished and protected her rest and mama-baby time; this was her core guardian at work. When a woman accesses her core guardian, she cares for herself in a more sustainable and satisfying way. Remembering what is most valuable to her, she focuses her attention there first—doing more only if her energy allows. By listening to her root guardian on a daily basis, Sarah will know if she has the energy to give or whether to simply retreat with her baby and focus on the heart of her mothering.

## Excess Vaginal Protection

Another pattern of energetic imbalance in the vagina is excess vaginal protection. This vaginal imbalance results in a high level of muscle guarding (excess muscle tension), making it difficult for a woman to receive the energy and nurturance necessary to sustain herself. This imbalance also creates a sense of isolation and scarcity.

Physical symptoms of excess vaginal protection include core muscle tension, trigger points in the muscles, and tightness. Vaginal tension may make pelvic penetration painful during sex, pelvic exams, or tampon insertion. Sometimes a woman has no awareness of pelvic pain or other outward signs of vaginal muscle tension, but she has multiple trigger points that can be felt by touching the pelvic muscles just inside her vagina.

Vaginal tension caused by this energetic imbalance is often mistaken for strength, because the tension is perceived as tone. However, a woman with this pattern will have difficulty engaging her pelvic muscles, and the vagina will have a hot sensation, indicating muscle distress and energetic stagnation. This woman may also experience urine leakage, constipation, hemorrhoids, or other symptoms of pelvic imbalance because her vaginal muscles are continuously tight and guarding, rather than providing a base of support. Reflections regarding excess vaginal protection include:

Have you ever had to protect yourself during an overwhelming experience?

Are you still guarding yourself at a high level?

What does your root voice say?

What support will enable you to release core tension and
restore pelvic balance?

### Women's Stories: Letting Down the Guard

Lara came for pelvic work to address vaginal discomfort. She
mentioned that she often felt guarded and on edge. She had some
history of abuse, which she had worked on with a counselor
to process her emotions. Now she wanted to feel more at ease
in her body and be able to enjoy lovemaking with her partner.

Lara's pelvic muscles had a high level of tension and many
areas of tenderness. Her muscles had increased their guarding
in response to previously unsafe situations. This high level of
pelvic guarding became her norm. However, the female body
can also respond to feeling unsafe by relinquishing the ability
to protect itself; this creates a vaginal imbalance of excess
receptivity. When this imbalance occurs, a woman is scarcely
present in her center, and her pelvic floor will have decreased
tone and areas of numbness. Both situations inhibit a woman's
connection to her body or ability to engage her chosen partner
with full satisfaction.

Respectful sexual exchange nourishes and balances the
female body physically and energetically. It was clear to Lara
that her past pelvic wounds were blocking her from receiving
this nourishment. However, less overt wounds may also block
partners from receiving one another in a nourishing manner.
By bringing her conscious presence to the pelvic space, a
woman can work with her pelvic wounds to be able to receive
sustenance when making love with a partner.

Lara wanted to address her vaginal imbalance and increase her receptivity. I taught her a breathing exercise to relax her musculature during the vaginal massage, but she needed to continuously remind her body that it was safe to let down its guard. Using a combination of hands-on pelvic work and visualizations, Lara was able to clear the energy of her pelvic space.

Initially, as Lara focused on her pelvic bowl, she felt a great divide between her upper and lower body; her lower body felt like a foreign territory. It took courage to travel through the barrier between these areas. As she brought her consciousness to her root again and again, Lara became more at ease in her pelvis. Her guarding energy decreased, and her vaginal muscles became more supple.

As Lara became more comfortable in her female body, she was able to reduce the overall tension in her pelvic muscles. As she increased her own awareness for and presence in the root, she felt less need to guard her root with patterns of holding. This change allowed Lara to experience her body and sexuality in a new way. Until now, sex had focused her attention on the part of herself most associated with danger and fear. As Lara inhabited more of her root, she felt peaceful in the core of herself. Sex became an opportunity to connect with her partner in an intimate space that now felt truly her own.

## Restore the Wild Feminine

A woman must address the imbalances in her vaginal energy to restore the wild feminine within herself. By accessing the full range of her vaginal energy, she restores the balance in her root as well as her ability to receive and protect the energy in her bowl. The qualities of both reception and protection are essential to a woman's health and enable her to cultivate the wild feminine in her core.

Vaginal imbalances associated with sexual abuse or other trauma may require skilled professional support from counselors, energy workers, or bodyworkers before physical or energetic balance is possible. Even without past abuse, a woman's pelvic wounds—from any kind of pain or shame associated with the female body—can block her sensuality or sexual intimacy. For example, past betrayals can affect her ability to let down her guard and inhabit the joyful aspects of her vaginal range. Fear and other doubts regarding feminine sensuality also restrict a woman's wild feminine expression.

Bring awareness to your vagina on a regular basis, noticing the patterns of receptivity and how it guards your root and life in general. A robust energetic presence in the pelvic bowl will allow you to cultivate and guard your creative energy. Instead of guarding with walls, that (inefficiently) block all types of energy, you attune with a vibrancy that supports health and repels or clears toxicity. Learn the sensations of your internal body to define where you are absent (sensations of numbness, cold, low energy, lack of awareness) and then restore presence (with breath, conscious attention, self-massage, the healing energy of spirit). Pay attention to your root voice to discover your body's unmet needs and desires. Replace all patterns of self-blame, shame, violation, and other limitations with the expansiveness of love in your center to free your sensual nature.

### Exercise: Vaginal Energy—Celebrating Your Root

1. Reflection: Ponder your relationship to your vagina and the ways you could celebrate this feminine ground. Notice how you have protected your female body or other things that you value. Examine where you have used your receptive powers. Reflect on how you desire to receive pleasure and express your sensual nature.

2. Ritual: Choose a color to represent your core vibrancy and wear it whenever you want to celebrate the full radiance of your root.

## Use Your Root Medicine

The root of the female body is precious. In the root, we can access our feminine intuition, this inner direction for our creative lives and for connecting our lives to spirit. The root holds our creative energy, our capacity for making a joyful life, but when we ignore or over-sexualize the root, we vastly diminish our access to the vibrant creative essence contained within our core. When we actively restore the range of the wild feminine—returning to the potential within ourselves to heal, create, and reinvent our lives—we make our own root medicine. We find the raw energy to heal the wounds of the feminine and build the structures that truly support our creative selves.

Root medicine is the wealth of healing resources that a woman learns in the process of restoring the physical and energetic balance to the root of her body. Over the years, while mothering my three sons, I have learned a whole array of holistic remedies for cuts, coughs, fevers, flus, rashes, and other ailments by working with their bodies. In the same way, as we explore even the most difficult regions of our feminine ground, we find some of our best and most potent medicine. This medicine can then be applied, like a supplement, to nourish a woman's daily vitality or used as a booster when she is particularly challenged or navigating a new part of her range.

I teach women to establish a solid presence in the root and make their basic root medicine through regular self-care: using vaginal massage, cultivating the energy flow of their ovaries and uterus, accessing their core creativity, and clearing the energy of the pelvic bowl. As a basic routine: vaginal massage one time per week, daily presence in the pelvic bowl to assist core energy balance, and added energy exercises as needed.

As she deepens her relationship with her body, a woman can modify her self-care as a way of living. During periods of high stress, she may add more vaginal massage to reduce physical tension. In times of transition, clearing the energy of her pelvic bowl or accessing the uterine energy several times per week will assist her process of transformation. If she is rejuvenating after a busy creative period, three to five days of cultivating the ovarian ability for nurturance and playful adventure will restore her core energy. By using root medicine to respond to her evolving needs, she renews her body's innate potential. Women who make and utilize their own root medicine are also better able to recognize and honor the root medicine of others, strengthening the community as a whole. Whether as specific self-care routines, rituals, energy tools, or other healing and creative works, the day-to-day development and application of root medicine enables us to change the nature of our lives as women.

When a woman is present in the root of her body on a daily basis, she is also present to receive the nourishment and inspiration available in every moment. She is able to address her needs as they arise and use her creative energy more efficiently, so there is more abundance in her life. Her wild feminine is at the ready whether she delves into the issues of her core or simply relishes the joy in her midst. Reflections to help you connect with your root medicine include:

What is your greatest source of stress or frustration?
How might you apply your root medicine to this part of your life?
What are your continuing inspirations and joys as a woman?
How might these relate to the making of your root medicine?

## Making Root Medicine: My Experience as a Creative Woman
The energetic patterns in a woman's root govern her use of creative energy. These patterns define what it means to be a woman, and

they determine her access to spirit and joy. They also shape her sensual expression and her capacity for tending her creations. The ways to change these patterns may differ from woman to woman, but as a woman learns about her most challenging patterns, she may also recognize the specific medicine in her root that will assist her in their transformation.

I discovered a current of rage running through my body—when I am upset, I go most easily to rage. From my compulsion to follow the path toward rage, I know this is a pattern from my lineage. When compelled to act or respond in a certain way, a woman is following a well-worn path, made trench-like by the actions of many who came before her. With the expression of rage, or with any other big emotional outburst, there is an accompanying emotional release. But the release does not resolve the deeper patterns. These underlying patterns cause energy to stagnate until pressure forces an outlet, and when energy is released in one great movement, rather than flowing out evenly, it sometimes causes more damage as it is expelled.

Exploring the channel that propels me toward rage, I have encountered the deeper patterns of self-denial and suppression that encourage a toxic buildup of energy. I have sensed the long line of women behind me: my ancestors and their hunger arising from generations of unmet needs and unrecognized potential. To get to these underlying patterns has required me to feel the rage in my body, but not to act on its energy. Instead of being swept along by a tide of rage, I turned inward, paying attention to the sensations of my root.

When the rage comes now, I slow myself down. I ask myself what is needed. Searching the tension in my body, I discover that I have gone too long without physical or spiritual sustenance. The emotional weight in my energy is suddenly unbearable. Rather than follow the rage or continue to ignore my internal struggle, I light a candle or make a bath for myself. I am aware of the bitter taste in my mouth. I feed myself and I pray. I work on the muscles of my root, massaging away the tension on my feminine side. I call on the assistance of spirit.

My root becomes tight and hot in the presence of my rage, and I feel disconnected from my body. In my bodily tension lies the compulsion to lash out and push away the comfort and nourishment I need. A simple action of self-care requires a monumental effort in the presence of my rage, but I make myself a bowl of soup, tell my partner how I am feeling, and take care of my needs. Nourishing myself while feeling the sensations beneath my rage offers external support as I begin to reroute the movement of this energy. Over time, I have made several, smaller, healing energy channels in my root for expressing my needs, taking breaks, loving myself, and using my energy sustainably to release the rage in a gentler manner. Following these energy channels has involved setting down everything that I thought needed to be done until I could reassess my priorities.

The most profound shift in my relationship with rage came from prioritizing my creative expression. Sometimes, while mothering my young children, I find a moment of peace between the chaos and the clutter. My first two children are playing quietly or at school, and the baby is napping; these are the productive windows of time where space opens and, if I choose to, I can accomplish the most tasks of the day. I could clean, I could organize; instead I leave every dirty dish or displaced toy where it stands and sit down to write. It feels delicious—and necessary—to put my creative needs first when otherwise I would be caught in an endless cycle of chores (like other women of my line). I make a cup of tea and I write. It is my daily delight.

I often finish a piece of writing, and then the baby wakes or my sons ask for a snack. If I had been working on household tasks, I would be angry at hearing another demand. I would believe that my needs could never be met and resent my children for it. But instead I feel an inner peace resulting from the mood of meditative reflection that arises as I write. My writing invites a direct connection with spirit that I can bring to the endless chores awaiting my attention. The load of daily household work is lighter when I have creative energy running through my body.

I have unearthed an internal rhythm of creativity that enriches my daily life as a mother. When acting from my root, I always have enough time and energy to write, take care of my children, and also restore some order to our home. It is a dance that might not work if I tried to place an external structure on my day. But by dropping into my writing when I sense the opening with my body, there is space for my creative expression that I would not have imagined in the midst of raising three children.

Living from my root provides an energy flow that serves my creative life. The rage still comes but much less often, and I have more resources to meet it. When I use my root in a particularly challenging moment, such as while feeling overwhelmed or exhausted by external demands, I am able to stay grounded and release pent-up energy in ways that are more gentle and manageable for my whole family. During these times of energy release, I might learn about another unmet need for the mothers of my lineage, one I must attend to for myself, in order to expand my creative range. With a regular movement of this energy, I recognize the fierce determination and burning passion that ties the women of my line together. When rage comes, I recognize the presence of a teacher and the opportunity to reclaim more range. With a daily creative flow, my range is no longer defined by rage.

When you desire to change your creative range, look for your most challenging patterns or unsustainable ways of using your creative energy. These may include denying your bodily needs, working without rest, addictive behaviors that drain your energy, or extreme emotions signaling a major imbalance in your core. You may feel compelled to follow a certain pattern, as if trapped or driven by an external force; these are the root patterns responsible for draining your creative energy. When you take direction from your root and make the medicine to heal these deep patterns that are stealing your vital force, you will realize your greatest potential as a creative woman.

### Exercise: Making Your Root Medicine

Call to mind a pattern that repeatedly challenges you. Because these patterns are often formed in response to losses or feminine wounding in your lineage, the regions where these patterns exist may feel like never-ending territory. Imagine them belonging to a beautiful piece of land that you inherited but never knew existed. When it is carefully cultivated, you may grow your best and most nourishing crop. This exercise will help you to make your root medicine and create a plan of action to use the next time this challenging pattern arises.

1. Call to mind the particular challenge and notice how your body feels; acknowledge the sensations of your root. Where does your energy flow, and where is it becoming blocked? Do you notice any tension, feelings of heat or cold, or any other sensations? How are you compelled to move? The next time you experience this challenge, try to slow down and pay attention to what is happening in your body. Move yourself in a direction away from the compulsion. Ponder your underlying or unmet needs.

2. Ask your body for two nourishing actions to assist your energy flow and restore core balance even in the midst of this pattern. Choose a quick action, in case time is short, and one that may require more time. When this pattern is triggered by a situation or event, begin your gesture of self-nourishment

and notice what happens. Pay attention to your body, especially your root. Feelings may arise, forms of resistance may appear; but focus on nourishing yourself, meeting your needs, and noticing your body sensations.

3. Your body is elemental and responds to the elements. Think of the elements you will have at hand, and use them to support your body's energy flow and to expand beyond your previous range. For example: having a warm cup of tea or taking a hot bath adds water to move emotions and the element fire, in the form of heat, to invigorate the energy system that is tending toward stagnation. Gazing at the sky brings air to clear mental patterns and inspires the spirit. Touch from another, a soft blanket, or a beloved animal brings the grounding earth element to restore your sense of tranquility. Use your root medicine to balance your body's energy flow and change the patterns in your core.

4. Observe the energy moving in your root for as long as you are able. If time is short, come back to this process later or make more of your root medicine the next occasion that this pattern arises. Reflect on any further assistance you may need: acupuncture, counseling, energy work, bodywork, a creative outlet, time spent in the wild, and so on, to strengthen your medicine. If you use this process whenever your greatest challenges arise, you will find that, step by step, you make your root medicine and recover previously inaccessible aspects of your range.

## Listen to the Root

When you listen to the root, even the most difficult situations can provide inspiration. Simply bringing your presence to the root is healing and offers guidance for how to restore and strengthen patterns that support core balance. Whether you are actively creating something or are in the midst of a challenging moment, use the following suggestions to increase your ability to listen from this wise place within yourself:

### Keys for Listening to the Root

1. Go within: Find your new direction from an internal place rather than responding to the outer circumstances.

2. Clear core tension: Use either hands-on massage or directed breathing to clear your core and receive your root wisdom with more clarity.

3. Set an intention: Make a clear statement about what you want in the present moment rather than reacting in some way.

4. Identify any needs: Take care of yourself and restore balance in your center. Focus your attention on meeting your true needs and desires.

5. Step outside or use the elements (air, fire, water, earth): Disengage from any reactive patterns and use the elements to encourage your core energy balance and flow.

6. Call on spirit: Say a simple prayer, light a candle, and open your energy to receive the divine support within and around you.

7. Nourish yourself: Encourage your ability to listen to the root by knowing how to give yourself nourishment and other acts of love and self-care.

## Tell Your Story, Find Your Path

This book is full of women's stories. Tell your own story of womanhood and you will find your path for restoring the wild feminine. Tell the story of your female body, your pride and your pain, and you will encounter the places in your life for celebration and healing. Speak about your lineage, its gifts and wounds, to continue the work of your ancestors. Examine your life as a whole, both in its areas of comfort and of challenge, to make your own way as a woman.

There is a natural tendency to turn away from or hide your wounds. You may not want to expose the vulnerable aspects of yourself. Yet, telling the story of your wounds takes away some of their power. It allows you to notice how they are influencing you and where they may be restricting your energy and your joy.

Begin to think of your wounds as your greatest assets. They are not a source of shame, but rather the soil for cultivating your potential. Each painful emotion or particular struggle that arises, revealing a place of wounding, will teach you the skills necessary to reap a bountiful harvest. Your wounds contain the knowledge you need to access your gifts, and as you claim even the difficult aspects of your experiences, you spend less energy avoiding parts of your range and more energy celebrating what you have gained.

Along the way, you find a greater ability to create what you want for yourself. Still, your journey will not be over. Blockages and other challenges continue to appear. This is not a sign of failure, but rather of growth. Your spirit is expanding, your capacity has increased, and so your path continues to evolve. Each time you restore balance in your pelvic bowl after an emotional storm or a physical crisis, you strengthen your core and your body's ability to find balance. Receive each challenge for what it is: an opportunity to reinforce or rebuild another aspect of your core patterning in order to sustain a vibrant and creative life. Doing this work is not an attempt to achieve perfection, but rather it is a dynamic process that reveals the real and authentic expression of your wild feminine self. Reflect on the story of your wounds with these questions:

> What are your deepest wounds as a woman?
> What stories do they tell?
> How would you like to transform these influences?
> What recent challenges are teaching you about new aspects of your creative range?

## Pelvic Wounds

Your pelvic space holds many of the wounds that you carry as a woman. It also contains the potential for your greatest transformation. It is important to speak of and heal pelvic wounds not only to access our own feminine gifts, but also to prevent a cycle of wounding from continuing into the next generation.

### Women's Stories: Claiming Her Fertile Ground

Laila came for pelvic work to increase her connection to this part of her body. She had tried to do pelvic muscle exercises but could hardly feel anything happening, and she noted that the women in her family completely ignored the female part of their bodies. She was ready to change this pattern.

Laila's pelvic muscles were extremely tense, with many painful places. As I began to massage away the tension in her muscles, tears welled in her eyes. I asked if working on her pelvic bowl was bringing up emotions, and she shared more of her story. Laila had been through extensive fertility treatments and had never conceived a child. The pain and disappointment were vivid even though the treatments had taken place over a decade ago. She had two daughters by adoption and felt content about her family. Still, she was surprised by the pent-up emotion that she found in working on her root.

I continued to massage Laila's pelvic muscles and encouraged her to breathe into her pelvic bowl. I invited her to let the healing tears flow and allow her grief its expression, and I talked to her about the importance of a woman's uterus for mothering her children. If she acknowledges this capacity in her core, an adoptive mother can hold her children energetically from her pelvic bowl just as a birth mother does. Laila's uterus was essential for nourishing her family and other heartfelt creations. As her children grew, she would be able to continue offering them energetic support by visualizing each one held in her pelvic bowl.

As we worked, more of Laila's energy returned to her core. She realized that she had dealt with her pain by avoiding this part of her body, and she also recognized a feeling of shame in relation to her body. Hearing the word infertile had made her feel unfeminine and as if her female body had failed in some way. She also remembered that both her mother and grandmother had had difficulty conceiving and had experienced multiple miscarriages; she knew that in their time it was considered important to be able to have large families. These family pressures and expectations about having children only added to Laila's sense of failure.

As she connected her feelings with her body sensations, her pelvic tension decreased. She also felt a sense of relief and renewed energy after clearing the emotional energy she had been holding. Laila came for several more sessions, and each time her pelvic muscle tension and pain was significantly reduced. By the last session, her symptoms were almost totally resolved and she had learned pelvic self-care tools to maintain her new pattern of pelvic health. Laila told me that she was proud to be the first woman in her family to claim her feminine creativity for her own intents and purposes.

As Laila told the story of her pelvic wounds, she was able to discover where she had given up her feminine ground. Identifying herself with the word infertile had diminished her sense of herself as a woman. This pain was exacerbated by a family who defined a woman's value by her ability to have children. Any woman who falls outside the boundaries of a family pattern of expectation may feel she has failed or that her expression of womanhood is not valued, and when a woman believes she has failed at womanhood itself, she often abandons her root, the place of her failure. In doing so, she also relinquishes essential creative potential. But if instead she changes her inherited pattern at its body level, by recognizing the inherent fertility in her female body that can be used to create and nourish what she herself values, she regains and even takes charge of her creative capacity. In this way, Laila was able to reclaim the fertile ground of her body.

Each wound that has marked your female body or feminine nature has a story that is relevant for you as a woman. Each story told will allow you to recognize what was lost or needs to be restored. As you bring to light patterns of wounding and transform their impact on your core, it is helpful to bless and clear your energy to support this change. Use the following exercise—inspired by traditional healer Rosita Arvigo and her book *Spiritual Bathing*—to clarify the energy around your body and home.

### Exercise: Making a Spiritual Bath

1. Fill a bowl with water. Gather some leaves or flowers, particularly from those plants that you are drawn to—aromatic herbs and roses are always good choices. As you gather the plant material, say a prayer asking in your own way for divine assistance. One at a time, place a flower petal or leaf into the water.

2. When you have finished gathering, look at the beauty created in this bowl. Notice the way each petal or leaf brings a color or shape to the water, just as your pelvic wounds and other experiences have touched and shaped your pelvic bowl.

3. Using your hands, squeeze the plant material into the water while saying a prayer. Ask for the healing, protection, or blessing that is needed. As Rosita, in passing on the teachings of Maya healer Don Elijio, has shared: *Trust with all of your heart that the healing will come to you.* Ask your root what else may assist the process of reclaiming the energy of your bowl. Take a moment for silence.

4. Dip your fingers into the water and moisten the skin over your womb, blessing your pelvic bowl. Bless any other areas of your body that are calling to you. Using your wet fingertips, splash the air around your body (like a bird taking a bath) to clear your energy field. Imagine this blessing extending out into your wild feminine landscape to brighten all the energy that radiates from or comes into your center, touching others in your circle as well. Sprinkle the water around your home, clarifying the energy of each room. Sprinkle family members and pets if you feel the impulse.

5. Pour this plant water onto the ground, giving thanks for the potential of regeneration present in your body, just as is held within the earth.

**A Purpose in Pelvic Wounds**
I have witnessed the changes in the female body when a woman acknowledges her pelvic or feminine wounds. One woman's uterus lifted several inches when she recognized the grief she was holding. Another woman's uterus pulled to one side as she described a

challenging situation in her life, then straightened as she named her frustrations and sense of powerlessness. The root muscles often begin to pulse as women identify core issues and release pelvic tension, allowing the return of energy and enhanced blood flow to the pelvic bowl.

As you come to know what wounds and strengths you hold in your center, your body no longer has to bear the weight of unrecognized burdens. The energy of your pelvic bowl becomes clear. With this new lightness in your body, you can feel the power, spirit, and joy of your creative fire.

The energetic patterns in your pelvic space reflect your beliefs about being female. You may be liberated in your mind, but your creative essence is still governed by the energy patterns of your pelvic bowl. When you look at your feminine wounds and your pelvic energy imbalances, you will discover how to realign your creative essence with your authentic nature. The energetic and physical changes that you make in your core will positively affect your whole creative capacity, changing your ability to draw energy in and manifest it in the form you desire.

Pelvic wounds can reflect grief associated with your female body and femininity; they can also be actual physical places where pain arises in your vagina and pelvic muscles. Pay attention to the way these wounds guide you to unclaimed aspects of your creative center. For example, you may periodically notice a painful area in the muscles of your vagina. If you have already addressed the mental or emotional associations regarding this wound, try incorporating vaginal massage or organ energy exercises to revitalize this region of your female body. Or look for lineage patterns that block your potential and begin to focus your healing work on the way these patterns are carried within your core.

Pelvic imbalances often arise in regions of the body that are already vulnerable because of muscle tension, decreased energetic presence, and less blood flow to the regions containing wound patterns. Recurring pelvic symptoms, like pain or tension in a particular area, signal the need for a holistic approach. When you experience recurring pelvic symptoms of physical or energetic imbalance, notice what is absent there. Ask your root what is needed in the place of this wound. Speak what was unsaid; identify and reclaim what was lost. Restore your awareness and energy to this part of your core, address any emotional burdens, and balance the masculine and feminine energies. Allow yourself to receive a blessing in this wounded place. Rather than simply trying to be rid of a particular block, reconnect with a region of wounding using thoughts, words, prayers, touch, trusted healers, and actions of love and respect.

Let the energy of your root move, inspire, and guide you to a healing response. Everything you need to know in order to do this is there in the resources of the pelvic bowl. Ask these questions about your most profound pelvic wounds:

What is this pelvic symptom or wound pattern drawing your attention to?

Which parts of your feminine (or masculine) range have yet to be addressed to transform the energy of this wound?

What imbalances in your body or daily life are preventing resolution of this pelvic wound?

How can you move your core energy and make a salve for this wound?

## Restoring a Joyful Sexuality

A woman needs to feel comfortable and secure with her body, the sexual energy in herself, and the sexual energy of her partner in order to experience a joyful sexuality. Many women have come to me for pelvic care hoping it will assist them to address a wounded sexuality. When a woman's sexuality is wounded, she is unable to be wholly present in her body or to fully receive the nourishment from consensual sex.

During engaged, healthy sex, both partners are emotionally present and respectful. They are more likely to be trusting and vulnerable with one another and to experience the beauty of their intimacy. When a woman or man has experienced early boundary violations, and other physical, emotional, or energetic traumas, the foundation of his or her sexuality becomes damaged. Depending on a person's age and the impact of a wounding experience, even one disruption can have significant effects. However, with the right attention and care, this damage can be repaired and a vibrant sexuality restored.

I have worked with women who participated in the sexual revolution of the sixties and who thought they were liberating their sexuality by having sex with multiple partners. But because they were typically disconnected from their roots while having indiscriminate sex, their bodies often felt violated. Though a woman may only recognize the extent of a violation or wound many years later, working with the energy of her pelvic bowl will bring the necessary healing.

Being uninhibited is not the foundation of a healthy sexuality (sometimes what is labeled as inhibition is really the guarding energy of the vagina alerting a woman to her sense of compromised safety). Rather, the core of healthy sexuality is full presence in your body and your connection with another person.

## Women's Stories: Rediscovering Her Own Desires

Cathy came for pelvic work to address her sexuality. She had been married previously to a partner who did not cherish her, and she often felt inhibited in their sexual connection. Cathy was dating again and met someone with whom she wanted to explore new patterns of intimacy, but she sought healing to assist this process.

As I began to work on Cathy's body, the first pattern in her bowl was related to grief. I encouraged her to notice the heaviness in her center and allow this energy to move. She recognized grief for her failed relationship, but even more so for being with a partner who was dishonoring and inattentive to her needs. Cathy had worked with a counselor to address the pain of her previous marriage, and now she began to clear the energy of this relationship from her body.

To heal the wounds inhibiting a full sexual connection, I encourage a woman to rediscover an intimate relationship with the root of her own body—just for herself—rather than focusing on her relationship to a partner. Doing so may require that she clear stagnant energy and acknowledge the emotions held in her bowl. Then she can focus directly on her own places of disconnection or blockage, places that can be the most difficult to acknowledge but also provide the most profound change. Overcoming sexual disconnection in this way can cause some personal discomfort because it requires focusing solely on oneself. But it also provides freedom from being defined by the perspective of a partner, who may only be a reflection of a woman's imbalance in her bowl and lack of her own self-cherishing. If she will heal the relationship with her body, first with herself, then she can continue with a loving partner to transform her presence in the pelvic bowl and experience a more fulfilling sexual connection. As a woman realigns with her own beauty, she will either find a new partner to celebrate and make love with or find that her current partner is responding to the shift in her center.

In Cathy's situation, she felt a sense of detachment from her root, almost as if she had given up on her sexuality, so I asked her to pay attention to the qualities of this disconnection. She saw an image of herself as playful and sexy, but it was far away, like it did not belong to her. Pondering her past marriage, Cathy realized that she felt confined in her self-expression, and she was relieved to release these constraints. Making this connection, she felt a tremendous heat begin to move through her pelvis. By focusing her awareness on the sensations in her core, she was healing the disruption and recovering her own intimate relationship with her body. By sharing this newfound intimacy with a respectful partner, she would further heal and expand this sensual part of her nature.

## Sex and the Body

Renew your relationship with your body and you will bask in your own radiance and delight in your senses. When you establish solid new connections to your tender, beautiful, wild root, you will find connection with your partner. Your sexuality may feel luscious or raw, passionate or vulnerable, as many expressions as you have in your root. When you experience the essence of your partner in this way, while fully engaged in your root, the energy of your bodies is exchanged in a profound and often healing manner.

Sex is a physical, emotional, energetic, and potentially spiritual event. Look to the areas where your sexuality is restricted to understand where your wild feminine feels unsafe. It is possible to have physical intercourse and be shut down emotionally during the process. Likewise, it is possible to share emotional intimacy but be terrified to express your physical desires with your partner. When you feel and respond from your root, you discover how your energy flows or becomes blocked.

Your sexuality is another place to encounter and heal your pelvic wounds, and be witnessed by the presence of another. Clarify the energy in your core by using your womb's natural rhythm of holding and releasing—you may shed the sexual energy that no longer serves you and retain the energy that nurtures your sexuality. Restore the full energy flow of your body and feel the passion of exchanging this energy with another. With compassion and curiosity, explore your wild feminine range with your lover.

If you (or one of your family members) was sexually violated in the past, your energy system may be frozen in a protective response, such as increased vaginal guarding, a closed left receptive ovary, or dissociation from the pelvic space. Sometimes the protective response is from direct experience, and other times it is simply inherited (from a lineage imprint) as a physical and energetic holding pattern. Although it is protective in nature, continuing to live with an energy response to violation in your core will prevent you from experiencing the joy of your sexuality as an adult. If your pelvic bowl still holds the effects of past sexual trauma, your root will need hands-on assistance to change core patterns and reflect what your mind already knows: you are now safe (safe to be here and safe to be radiant).

Use vaginal massage to address the tension in your muscles. Remind your vagina to let down its guard. Breathe into your ovaries to create pelvic boundaries (strengthening your ability to choose what you receive into yourself) and then allow yourself to feel the energy of your partner. If you experience overwhelming emotions, take a break or enlist the help of a counselor. This is your root, and you have the right to experience the pleasure of meeting your chosen one here.

Being able to feel pleasure is a gauge of your root connection. Working with your root, you can begin to explore your own sensations of pleasure. Doing vaginal massage will increase the health of your muscles, enhancing sexual enjoyment and your potential for orgasms because both require ample blood and energy flow as well as good alignment and muscle tone. But the deepest aspects of pleasure also require an energetic wholeness where your own spirit and body meet. Working with your root connection will guide your path toward wholeness.

## Personal Wounds, Universal Healing

Having watched women reclaim the feminine in their bodies and personal lives has led me to believe that each woman has a role in restoring a universal connection to the feminine (and with it a more playful and robust masculine). As each act of courage—including being able to cherish ourselves and take pleasure in our feminine qualities—challenges limiting aspects of femininity, a greater range of creative potential is recovered for the whole community. As women share their stories with each other, they recognize their own part in this larger process.

Stories inform our sense of what is possible as women. They have the potential to heal, because in their telling, the truth often unfolds. Stories teach us that we are not alone and that we can change patterns of abuse and domination. When we use stories to heal these wounds, we not only transform ourselves but we change the path for all women. Untold stories still exist under the surface of our consciousness, influencing the meaning of womanhood. But it is in the telling that a story's medicine is made manifest, available for all who listen to partake.

## Root Medicine and Transformative Acts

While pregnant with my second son, I received a deeper under-standing of feminine wounding in my family and in our culture in general. I dreamed one night that I was surrounded by a circle of women. In the dream, I was pregnant and draped in elaborate scarves and jewels. I felt like a goddess, celebrated and feminine. When I shared the dream with a friend of mine from India, she told me that it sounded like the ritual performed in her country for every pregnant woman because it is believed that, while pregnant, a woman is a goddess incarnate. Because she is carrying the divine during her pregnancy, people come to receive her blessings.

Hearing the words of my friend, I felt a deep longing. My own culture, obsessed with beauty in the form of a thin, almost anorexic, female body, was unsatisfying. Most parenting magazines prescribe workouts for women to recover their pre-pregnancy shape and offer a wealth of other shallow advice regarding the female body.

My own pregnant body felt ripe and sensuous, earthy and holy. Having given birth already, I loved the way that birth opened my womb and vagina. I felt alive in my root and had no desire to return to some other form. The idea of being celebrated as a goddess enlivened every cell in my body; this would be a way to soothe generations of pregnant woman who were unrecognized or even shamed as their bodies sheltered another life.

My friend and I created a ritual to honor this pregnancy, based on my dream and her cultural knowledge. I invited a group of women to gather in my home. On the day of our gathering, my friend pinned a piece of vibrant yellow silk to my hair that fell across both shoulders. I wore a silk skirt beneath my bulging belly, but left my belly bare. I had jewels around my neck and bangles on my arms. Aside from the day of my wedding, it was the most radiant I have ever felt.

During the ritual, I knelt before each woman saying, "I honor the feminine in you." Then each woman came forward and said the same words to me and to my unborn baby. My friend placed a special red powder on my forehead and belly. Another friend took photographs, capturing the changing and intensifying light in the room as our ritual progressed. It was as if my baby and I were bathed in gold, a halo of light outlining my pregnant form.

This ritual was my own way to address patterns of wounding regarding the feminine in my lineage. Both genders have suffered consequences from the degradation of the feminine, and I became aware of this pain in myself because I was attuned to the child growing in my womb. Rather than attempting to shield my child, I used my root medicine to form a ritual, answering the call for healing that arose from the center of my being.

People asked me if I chose to honor the feminine because I thought that I was having a girl. But to me, the gender of my child was irrelevant. The feminine belongs to girls *and boys*, women *and men*. The feminine is an essence, not a gender: whoever understands this, also understands the feminine.

## What about the Men?

Tapping into the profound nature of the pelvic bowl, women ask me, "What about the men?" It is true that men also have a sacred center which has often been misunderstood or neglected, compromising their energetic and physical potential. Their pelvic bowls are also in need of better care, with organ energies that relate to their creative essence. And since they were an egg in their mother's ovary and gestated in her womb, the information in *Wild Feminine* relates to them as well. There are pioneers working in the field of male and female pelvic health, including Jean-Pierre Barral, a French osteopath whose visceral manipulation bodywork is studied around the world and who has developed skilled manual therapy techniques for the prostate. More awareness for the importance of pelvic work in male health will assist men in receiving this type of care.

As the mother of three sons, I also recognize the vital importance of feminine energy in their lives, for nurturing an active creativity and developing a robust and authentic masculine. To support their relationship with the feminine, I have encouraged them to play music, create with their hands, spend time in the natural world, pay attention to and take care of their bodies, understand the value of *being* in relationship to *doing*, and live with an awareness for internal energy flow and creative cycles—to know their own beauty. Male access to the feminine, whether as sons, partners, brothers, or friends, is also greatly enhanced as women restore their bodily relationship to the feminine. With a revived feminine, the next shift will arise in new forms of the masculine.

## Working from the Root

As women, we do our best work when we draw upon the wisdom of the root. I always encourage my clients to pay attention to the root whether they are balancing the energy of the pelvic bowl, accessing their creativity for a particular project, or exploring new ways to nurture themselves and mother their children.

One of my clients took this approach to her job as a nurse in a large hospital. After learning about how to access her root in a bodywork session, she was inspired to write *Work from the Root* on the top of her clipboard before making her nursing rounds. These words reminded her to respond from her core while interacting with her patients. She found that she acted from a place that was deeper and more satisfying—for herself as well as for the patients who received her care. Imagine the range of expression for the wild feminine when women from all walks of life begin to work from their roots.

### Keys for Working from the Root

- Make space for daily reflection to receive the insights of your body and promptings from spirit.
- Clear any physical, emotional, mental, or spiritual blocks that limit your self-nourishment, and simultaneously create structures and living practices (in these same realms) that sustain you.
- Regularly express the beauty and playfulness of your creative essence.
- Move and create from an internal place: ask yourself how you are inspired to create, what you need, what you are drawn to.
- Set creative intentions in both monthly and annual rituals to actively cultivate your creative rhythms.
- Find opportunities for daily delight: music, color, laughter, poetry, children, friends, food, nature, prayer, and so on.
- Seek your joy: go toward whatever uplifts your spirit.
- Expand your sensual nature: touch with full presence; attend to your sensations; notice where energy and the body meet and spirit becomes form.

When you work from the root in all aspects of your life, you discover the true potential of your female body. Whatever question, struggle, or desire you have within yourself—work with it from the root. No longer limited by the wounds you encounter in your pelvic bowl, you apply your own root medicine. Ultimately this root medicine is your most essential creation because it will restore the flow of joy—the joy in your female body, the joy in your daily life, and the joy for all those who are nourished from your bowl.

## Joy: Celebrate Your Wild Femininity

Your female body is a place of joy and miracles. This is the birthplace of all future children—universal and yet uniquely personal. It defines your feminine ground and houses your sensual desires. It contains unlimited creative potential and connects you to a shared sister-hood of women. Your root wisdom is here, an ancient knowing that arises from the ebb and flow of your womb. Celebrate your wild femininity: this being a precious gift.

Joy does not equate to happiness, although it has an expansive-ness that invites delight. Joy is being able to settle completely into the sensations of a given moment and receive the fullness of the blessing it contains. It is a practice of self-love, feeling worthy of and connected to the beauty of life. We can increase our capacity for joy by working with the energy flow and tension patterns of the root. It is by attuning to the root that we find—and experience—our joy.

### The Root Voice of Joy: Fierce Grace

As you listen to your root voice of joy, your health will be restored. Vaginas feel joyful when nurtured; they love baths and warm air. They like to dance and celebrate being alive. If you are listening to your joyful root voice, you will take naps and eat good food. You will tell stories and laugh out loud. You will tickle your children and sing songs with them. You will indulge your senses and sleep well. You will honor yourself because you know your value as a woman. You hear the voice that says, *I am woman, hear me roar.*

When I first began working on my own root, I could conceive of joy but had no way to feel it. As the energy returned to my core, the sensations of joy were rekindled in my body. I more readily joined the boisterous joy of my sons as I cleared my root tension. In finding your own root voice of joy, you rejuvenate and give sustenance to your spirit. You recalibrate your body to run on the energy of joy—and this energy now flows more easily into all aspects of your life.

### Exercise: Celebrating Your Joy with a Blessing Stick

1. Reflection: Ponder your greatest creative joy. Notice where you feel it in your body. Explore the sensations of joy. Imagine how you would like to bring this feeling into the various regions of your body and life.

2. Ritual: Make a blessing stick for yourself or with a group (this process is similar to the grief ritual on page 191). Gather strips of paper, a medium-size stick, and string. Take a moment to reflect upon your hopes, dreams, prayers, and joys and then write about them. If you are making the stick for yourself, write on individual slips of paper. When you are finished writing, tie these papers to your stick while sensing the expansive energy that arises when you reflect upon joy, creative dreams, and gratitude. If you are in a group, invite each individual to reflect inwardly, and then have each person write about these reflections on their own piece of paper. When finished, each person ties their paper onto a collective stick. Then place the stick onto an altar, into a body of water, into the earth, or onto a fire to release this energy to spirit. Whether in solitude or with a community, encourage your wild feminine to roam in this expansive range of your joy.

*Note: A blessing stick makes a wonderful gift to celebrate some-one, assist in healing, or mark a transition in some way. Invite members of the community to write blessings and wishes for this individual, collectively creating a blessing stick.*

If a woman forgets her joy, she will often work too hard and restrict her intake of rest and food. She will begin to measure her worth according to the standards of those outside herself or by what she produces, which is never enough. She will be tired and tense and disconnected from her authentic being. Working among societal constructs that do not support the wild feminine, she will reflect the predominant culture, which values productivity and quantity over sustenance and quality.

If, instead, a woman follows the voice of her root, which con-nects her to the source of her joy, she has abundant capacity to nourish herself and all her creations. She cherishes herself and knows her intrinsic worth. She expands the notion of what it means to be a woman, giving form to her dreams, celebrating along the way. Further reflections on joy include:

Where in your body and life does your joy flow freely?
Where do you block or lose touch with joy?
What is needed to bring back your joy in these regions?
How can you support joy in your daughters or sons and the other women and men guiding our future?

*Women's Stories: Witnessing Her Radiance*

Jean came for pelvic work to support her healing after two miscarriages. When I asked her to bring attention to her pelvic space, she began to visualize her inner pelvis and said she saw a golden light all around her uterus. This surprised her because her primary association with her body was a sense of anger.

She felt angry and let down by her body for not carrying her pregnancies to term.

Jean visualized her womb space and found a radiant and luscious place. She realized that she had been completely disconnected from her pelvis and had not even noticed what her body was experiencing since the miscarriages. As Jean focused on her body sensations, she felt a weight lift: it was the burden of resentment she held against her body. This was related not only to her miscarriages, but to other hurtful experiences also associated with being female.

As Jean released these pent-up feelings from her womb, she described a sense of giving birth and a rush of energy in her body. The golden light around her womb expanded to fill her entire pelvic space, a newly fertile ground. Feeling the radiance of her womb, Jean reconnected with a sense of internal joy that she had forgotten long ago.

Spending time in the activities or places that bring you joy enables you to re-access the beauty of your feminine nature. Joy is a light energy enhancing the flow of your body and refueling your wild feminine spirit. Reflect further on your joy with these questions:

How do you presently express your joy?
What activities bring you effortless joy?
How do you share your radiant joy with others?

## Pay Attention to Your Root
The core physical and energetic patterns of your root can guide you toward restoring access to your full feminine range. Follow the instincts of your vagina regarding issues of intimacy, sexuality, feminine identity, and ownership of your female body, and connect

with your ovaries to nourish and claim your creative fire. Listen to your uterus to gestate and give birth to your heartfelt creations. Examine your fallopian tubes, the balance between your fiery ovaries and steadfast uterus, in relation to creative and intimate partnerships. Every aspect of your female body that calls your attention serves to reawaken your wild feminine spirit.

Know the signs of balance in your body: engaged pelvic floor muscles, ability to receive nourishment, active creative expression, sense of peace and relaxed muscles in the root, vibrant and balanced core energy, and ability to give and receive touch. These reaffirm the health of your daily routine. Be aware also of signs of imbalance in your body: tense or unengaged pelvic muscles, dampened sensation, depleted resources, decreased energy, stagnant creative expression, mood swings or excessive cravings, sense of being overwhelmed, and avoidance of touch or bodily needs. These symptoms signal your body's desire for change.

Look to the areas in your life you associate with wholeness in your female body, and you will find your strength. Seek the experiences of pain or loss involving your body, and you will encounter potential for transformation. Depending on your experiences with sexuality, the tendency to over-sexualize the female body may have caused you to block your root connection. As you discover where you have relinquished the vital connection to your root, you will find the path to reclaim your womanhood. One of my clients said that attending to her root was emotional. She remembered the pain of past relationships and pelvic exams, but now she finds hope in her body as well.

## Be Clear about Your Blocks

When your core creative energy is flowing, your joy flows easily. When there are emotional burdens and other energy blocks in your center, your creative flow is restricted and your channel for joy is constrained as well. But when a situation triggers one of your emotional burdens, such as a deep well of rage or grief that is out of proportion to the trigger, you have a golden opportunity. Though emotions are compelling, recognize the pain as deeper than the situation at hand. Resist the urge to blame someone else and instead look within for the clarity of your root. This is an emotional burden that is blocking your joy.

Feel the sensations of how this block is carried within your body for direction on how to move the energy in your core. If the sensation feels heavy, let yourself rest. If it feels tight and restricted, take a bath or a walk to assist your energy flow. If there is a sense of aggression or agitation, sit on the grounding earth or take some deep breaths to find your center. Nourish yourself, identify your needs, work on your root medicine, and be clear about your desire to rebuild core patterns, so they can easily channel joy. Even as we encounter challenges, we have a choice in the energy we hold as the following poem reminds us:

> Say yes to joy.
> No to all else.
> Yes to the people.
> No to the negative energy.
> Yes to yourself.
> Yes to the sacred.
> No to demands or despair.
> Yes to life.
> Yes to love.
> Yes to your beauty.
> Yes to yourself in joy.

## Cherish Your Female Form

Reflect on the nature of your female form. Your relationship to your body and your femininity will shape the range of your wild feminine. Ponder the creative range you desire for yourself, and rethink any negative associations regarding your female body or femininity. Identify anything that limits your ability to celebrate yourself as a woman. As you begin to cherish all aspects of your womanhood, you will discover more ways to access your authentic nature. Your real feminine form is like a beautiful gem, a multifaceted radiance. Sense the layers of beauty within color, music, nature, art—know that you are part of this beauty. Find new feminine associations by creating a wild feminine work of art.

### Exercise: Creating a Wild Feminine Work of Art

This exercise involves making a creation or personal expression about your radiance or relationship with the wild feminine. Begin by choosing a hands-on medium: paint, clay, collage, colored pencils, charcoal, and paper, or natural materials like stones, mud, sticks, and leaves. Then select a theme to inspire your creation. Create from your root rather than your head by following the creative inspirations that arise in the process (such as the shades, textures, or shapes you are drawn to rather than attempting to make something that "looks or sounds good") as you explore a particular theme. Themes may include the following or one of your own invention:

- Illustrate the essence of your beautiful, wise, angry, strong, wild, fearful, or sacred vagina/wild feminine.
- Make a model of your wild feminine landscape: the true shape of your full creative range.
- Make a healing work of art as salve for your feminine wounds.
- Make a piece inspired purely by your radiance.

For further inspiration, create another piece while focusing on the creative direction that arises from your womb, your ovaries, your whole pelvic bowl, the present state of your creative energy, the new forms you are making, or some additional aspect of your feminine or masculine nature. Notice how these works are similar or different as you change the focus of your awareness.

## Make Your Own Form

As inherently creative beings, it is part of our work to know our creative desires and make our own forms—these outward expressions of our creative energy that support our creative flow. There is no right way to be a creative woman; each decides for herself how she will express her creative essence. If you find that you have been holding the energy of others instead of building your own creations, then you may release their energy. As a woman, you have a tremendous creative capacity that belongs to you. You do not have to exchange anything to receive this potential.

Reclaim your innate creativity by loving and working with your root. You can be more vibrant, visible, and present—gathering energy from your whole wild feminine range. Whenever an existing form—a body pattern, way of being, defined role, daily habit, relationship dynamic—no longer serves you, it is time to make a new form. From the clarity of your center, notice where the energy is restricted. Use breath, visualization, organ energy, ritual, prayer, or specific direction from your root. Focus on what you want to create. Take up your rightful, powerful pelvic bowl, draw new energy resources from the greater realm of spirit, and make your own form.

### Exercise: Your Pelvic Bowl Sings

Do this exercise to enhance your creative capacity or find support in challenging moments. Your core resources are most accessible when there is harmony in your bowl.

1. Center: Find your center. Drop down to this internal creative place within yourself. Take note of how you are feeling in this space and sense the present state of your creative energy.

2. Clear: Clarify your bowl by sweeping the energy with your inner awareness. Give permission for your body to clear anything that no longer serves you. On each inhale of your breath, imagine fresh energy rejuvenating your center. With each exhale, invite a full release.

3. Balance: Balance the inner fire (feminine) and the outer fire (masculine) to move your creative flow in a dynamic and sustainable manner. Focus on your left ovary: invite your feminine radiance to nourish and inspire your center. Focus your right ovary: invite your masculine radiance to create new forms that protect and celebrate the feminine. Align these core fires within. Set your intentions in the womb space.

4. Bless: Call on the sacred to bless your center. Invite the brilliant radiance of spirit to fill your bowl. Relish this shimmering light; remember that you are sacred.

5. Sing: Take this vibration and engage your full capacity to live with joy and to embody your radiance. Meeting each ordinary or extraordinary moment from your center, your pelvic bowl sings.

**Honor Your Body**
Honor your female body. Do what it likes: dancing, hiking, napping, eating, or laughing. Bathe yourself with intention and care. Wear fabrics that appeal to your skin, colors that make you happy. In the cold, wrap a layer around your pelvis to warm your bowl. Thank your root for each creation and for the fire that enlivens your womanhood.

When your uterus is shedding its blood or you are in a mode of release, rest and spend more time in your home. Rub castor oil on your lower belly, just over your womb, and cover it with a warm cloth to assist your body in releasing from the core. To enhance your vibrancy, go out into the fresh air and let it soak into every cell. Place Epsom salts in your bath or go to the sauna to further reinvigorate your body, this house of your wild femininity.

### Exercise: Calling on the Elements

Your body is elemental. Use this blessing to call on the elements and bless your beautiful form:

> May I be like the blessed earth: growing, nourished, blossoming, grounded.
> May I be like the blessed water: flowing, clear, life-giving, free.
> May I be like the blessed fire: warm, radiant, tended, wild.
> May I be like the blessed air: light, open, inspired, essential.

## Let Yourself Be Held

The journey can be hard. Remember your connection to earth and spirit—and let yourself be held. May the following meditation assist you.

### Exercise: Mother Earth and Father Sky

1. Go and lie upon the earth.

2. Spread your body out and set down your weight. Notice the texture beneath you. Feel the depth of support that travels deep into the earth. Let your body rest against this tender ground.

3. Notice the presence beneath you, the energy and aliveness of the earth. Let yourself be held by this ancient presence, Mother Earth.

4. Now bring your awareness to the air and sky above. Feel the lightness that brushes your skin, the current that moves the branches of trees and carries the flight of butterflies and birds.

5. Listen for the sounds that are carried on the wind. Speak your prayers so they too may be carried. Feel the expanse of sky overhead and let it lift your spirit. Let yourself be inspired by this ancient presence, Father Sky.

6. Give thanks for Mother Earth and Father Sky, always here to hold you.

## Cry Out to Spirit

When you are navigating difficult regions or are in the midst of your own pain, cry your hopes and prayers out to spirit. Let yourself be open and vulnerable, sharing your most intimate self. Spirit is always there for us, but we often close ourselves off from this energy when we are hurting. You may call to spirit in prayer, in movement or song, in ritual, or as if speaking with a trusted friend. It is helpful to go outside or to do something that brings you in touch with the senses of your body. When I most need the company of spirit, I make a fire. I choose and shape the sticks as an expression of my present state, and then I add fire and watch the changing forms, the dance of wood and flame, and receive the blessing it contains.

## Remember Spirit in the Womb

We can find spirit in the womb. A woman's body is the doorway through which every person enters to begin her or his time here on earth. If we can remember this connection to spirit in the root of

the female body, we will also remember to honor the sacred in ourselves. We will clear the extraneous from our bodies and our lives,
leaving more room for our relationship with spirit.

When a woman comes to me with a question about her female
body, I do not give her an answer. I point her to her womb. All the
answers she needs about her children and her own creative purpose
are there in her womb, the beginning place. It is the source of new
life and the connection to the lives that came before us. A woman
will receive all she desires if she will go to the root and place her
trust in spirit there.

This individual connection radiates into the larger community.
First one woman remembers how to access spirit in her core, and
then another. The children of these women remain connected to the
sacred in themselves. And the partners of these women remember
their own sacred beginnings. This is the way the feminine returns.

### Exercise: The Sacred Pelvic Bowl

1. Bring your awareness to the womb space in the center of
   your pelvic bowl. Notice your breath in and out. This is your
   own place for receiving the intuitive wisdom, healing, or
   inspiration of any given moment.

2. Call to the four directions from within your bowl, noticing
   the response to each call:

   What is here for me in the front of my bowl?
   What is here for me to the right of my bowl?
   What is here for me behind my bowl?
   What is here for me to the left of my bowl?

3. Accept what you receive, realizing that by the simple act of
   calling out from your bowl in this way, you are opening

yourself to the vast energy resources of spirit. Close this exercise by saying, *With gratitude, I receive the blessings of my sacred pelvic bowl and the divine, helpful, and protective energies that surround me.*

## Ride the Sacred Wave

Doing this work—changing our relationship to the root of our bodies and the feminine within ourselves—is not to create and do more, but rather to know what it is that we already have. Our power is our presence. We discover the power within our bodies to be fully present with whatever happens to be in our path, right in this very moment. With our full presence in the root, we also find the sacred flow that is always there, and we move or create from this place. We can drop down into this greater flow, from our own center, to receive the support and healing, the inspiration and intuition, the comfort and blessings, all that spirit contains for us in the exact way that we need it. Joy is what we find, in the power of our presence and the company of spirit, riding this sacred wave.

## Follow Your Body toward Joy

My spirit soars whenever I go to the ocean. It has always been this way, and I take my sons to the edge of the sea whenever I want to share my understanding of joy. I often bring them to one particular beach along the Pacific coast.

One day I was on the phone with my mother, telling her about our day trips to this beach. She said that I was taking my sons to the same beach she had gone to as a child. Her mother took her there to visit her grandfather, who lived nearby at the time. Those days at that beach were some of her happiest childhood memories.

My earliest beginnings in my mother's body imprinted in me her sensation of joy at this beach along the Pacific Ocean. The joyful response of my body leads me back to the same beach as a grown woman. The body naturally moves us toward joy.

## Go to the Wild

Connect with the earth and the wild in your midst. Tend a piece of land, sift the dirt with your hands. Notice the layered ground and the way it shapes and sustains what grows. Lift your attention upward. Listen for the rush of bird wings or the rustle of leaves. See the vibrant shades of a flowering bush or the colors that spread across a morning sky and how they change with each touch of light.

Going to wild places, or paying attention to the wild around you, awakens the deep wild nature in your body. Recognizing that you are part of this landscape—inherently alive and wild—restores the flow of ancient energy currents, bringing the vital life force and infinite expression to your own inner landscape.

Reclaim your root and you will have everything you need as a woman. The experiences that previously diminished your feminine power now remind you how to hold your ground. The challenging aspects of your lineage offer inspiration for your work in life. The roles available to you as a female take on new shape and dimension. You embody a dynamic form. Your feminine self is a bold expression, every aspect your own creation. Making your root medicine, you encounter the mystery of spirit in your sacred pelvic bowl. You experience the joy that your smile reveals, the joy of a wild feminine who knows her range.

*May you know and love your beauty.*

# A Woman's Prayer

*I* am drumming. The sea stretches out before me and catches the sound of my drum. The soft sand holds me like a cupped hand. I have come to drum my thanks for all that I have been given. The beat of my drum is a prayer. I drum toward the sky. I drum toward the earth. I drum and feel the sound against my skin. The sound of my drum pounds against the resistance in my body that holds back the river of my joy.

I sit and drum as my husband and three sons explore the beach, their male bodies propelling them to move. My two oldest sons run back and forth in long arcs while my husband walks with a steady gait, our new baby son in his arms. I drum in the sand, watching the shapes made by their constant motion. My joy rises like a tide.

I close my eyes and lift my face to the sun. When I open my eyes again, the four males I journey with have come together. My eyes travel an expanse of sand to find them. The black outline of their bodies stands like a cairn, a stack of rocks carefully placed to call the spirit home.

I drum until joy flows through me like the light across the water. The edges of my resistance soften and I remember my pelvic bowl. I am returning to the root of my female body. I am seeking the heart of my feminine self. My root is my place of knowing. I come here to know myself. Roaming the land of the wild feminine, I am free. All is untamed and pure gold. I am just who I am. Daughter, mother, lover, teacher, healer, all my selves stand at the door and await my return. Surrounded by the curve of these bones, the walls of this womb, the light of these ovaries, I will sit in the peace of my body. I perch on the edge of this shining sea, spinning the thread of a woman's joy, drumming my wild self to spirit.

*Take your creative dreams.*
*Place them in the deeper currents,*
*Where your body meets spirit—*
*And they will become real.*

# Acknowledgments

With a grateful heart, I acknowledge the tremendous forces and individuals who came together to make this work possible. To spirit, for a bright and illuminating light. To the ancestors, my mother and father lines, I feel your presence. To the spirits of the land, I give thanks.

Thank you to all the women who have worked with the wild feminine in my workshops and in my practice—too many to name, together a force of nature. Each of you has offered your insights regarding root medicine or shared the healing and creative potential of your bodies directly. Your courage is an inspiration. If you have been touched by this work, you have contributed to bringing the root medicine into a tangible form. May you continue to receive the blessings of the wild feminine in your daily life.

Thanks to the writers and editors whose gifts with words and insights into the world of publishing were true blessings: Elizabeth Lesser, Ned Leavitt, Britta Alexander, Jean Hegland, Dan Imhoff, Kathy Glass, and Sara Guest.

Thank you to those who held a flame at critical times and kept my own creative fires burning: Carol Ferris, Howard Ludwig, Tina Lilly, Cindy Tenant, Padrice Stewart, Sohi McCaw, and Lainie Butler Kennedy.

To my teachers, a profound thank you for sharing your life's work to make the path possible: MJ Strauhal, Dr. Sheila Murphy, and more recently Rosita Arvigo.

To all the healing arts practitioners who have shared the potential of this work with others.

To Adrienne and Esme Fuson, for a direct touch from spirit. To all the baby spirits.

Thanks to the healers who have strengthened my form: Dr. Judith Boothby, Dr. Susan Allen, Elizabeth Zenger, and Joseph Soprani.

To Tom Spanbauer, neighbor and local inspiration, for breaking apart old forms and bringing in more beauty.

Thanks to my writing goddess and sister of the heart, Nancy Cook, and her womb light, Izi, for helping me make this fire.

To Liliana Barzola Read, bright star, for keeping the energy clear and in vibrant flow.

To John Livingston, for bringing in the angels and strengthening the protective energy field.

To my Portland mama friends, especially my book club, and the many mothers who grace my work, who know how to savor life and mothering.

Thanks to Kate Hass for editing and Timothy Rice for designing the beautiful and first *Wild Feminine* (self-published) book. To Susan Gross for fabulous cover art that continues to inspire.

Taking apart a book and reweaving it to an enhanced form was a truly joyful process with Beyond Words president and editor in chief Cynthia Black. Also thank you to Beyond Words publisher Richard Cohn and Atria Books publisher Judith Curr. I am particularly grateful for the blend of spirit and body that Beyond Words brings to publishing and for their cultivation of the wild feminine. A heartfelt thanks for the passion and talent of editorial and production staff: Jenefer Angell, Dan Frost, Lindsay S. Brown, Devon Smith, Ali McCart, Heather Jones, Emmalisa Sparrow, Whitney Quon, and Georgie Lewis.

Thanks to Jan Waldmann and Scott Mahood for loving books and taking care of this one.

Thanks to Dancing Crow for a beautiful ceremony to bless *Wild Feminine*.

Thank you to my family for laying the groundwork and creating my love of home: Glenn and Melodie Petry, Ruth and Bill Love, Cheri, Julie, Greg, and Vanessa.

To Jan and Darrell Kent for walking in integrity, solidly on this earth, and holding me as your own. To Sara, for our long-running thread that continues to weave its blessing.

To my sons, Nick, Gabe, and Japhy—your brilliant radiance ignites the joy. May you always know your beauty. Your wild masculine presence brings such balance and delight to each day.

To my spirit daughter Maia—here is my promise: your light shines on.

To my husband, favorite wordsmith, and love, Dan—your strength is a constant presence, a fire that enlivens my own. Thank you for co-creating with me and sharing a passion for the wild.

Thanks to Kiva, Blue Magoo, and Kona too.

And finally, I offer my deep gratitude to the wild feminine, for keeping me company through many dark nights and inspired days, winter and summer, nursing babies and tending children, and whispering words by the fire. You are loved.

# Appendix

## Starting a *Wild Feminine* Book Club

*T*here is power in gathering with women. We learn from and inspire one another, and our energy is enlivened by the circles we create. The wisdom of this book has been distilled from many women and will take on new forms and greater meaning in a community; as it is shared and discussed among women, it will evolve. This section offers seven discussions for a *Wild Feminine* book club. Each discussion, one for each chapter, contains overall themes, suggested readings, and activities to accompany each session. It is meant as a beginning, a place to meet the wild feminine together.

# Session 1: Landscape

**Readings:** Introduction: Coming Home, and Chapter 1: Beginning Your Journey

**Opening:** Read aloud the opening for chapter 1 to call together the energy. Do a brief check-in for each woman to share your intention for exploring this work.

**Group Discussion Questions:**

How do you relate to the wild feminine landscape (page 4)?
Where is the wild feminine visible in your life?
Where would you like to cultivate more connection with
    the wild feminine?

**Group Reflection:** Have one woman lead the group in the Visualizing the Pelvic Bowl exercise (page 15). Afterward, share what you noticed with one another regarding your own inner landscape.

**Group Activity:** Spend five to ten minutes pondering and then writing down three of your creative visions or dreams. With the group, share one of your creative dreams and how it relates to the range of your wild feminine. Take the paper with your three dream seeds home to either plant in your garden or place in a sacred space as an intent to nurture your heartfelt creations.

**Closing:** Read aloud the last paragraph in chapter 1 (page 28), and then close the gathering with a Circle Blessing: Form a circle and join hands. Each woman speaks a single word that comes to her as one of her hopes or prayers (either spontaneously or in relation to a particular theme). Go around the circle three times until each woman has given three words.

# Session 2: Body

**Readings:** Chapter 2: Exploring Your Feminine Ground

**Opening:** Read aloud the opening for chapter 2 (page 29) to call together the energy. Do a brief check-in for each woman to share what you have learned since the last gathering.

**Group Discussion Questions:**

What patterns do you notice in your female body?
How do these patterns shape the flow of your creative energy?
Where do you desire to restore pelvic balance or reclaim your creative ground?

**Group Reflection:** Have one woman lead the visualization as the group does the Clarifying the Energy of Your Bowl exercise (page 49). Afterward, share what you noticed regarding your pelvic energy.

**Group Activity:** Do the ritual part of the Honoring Your Pelvic Bowl exercise (page 39). As a group, share your desires for healing, celebration, or in some way enhancing your relationship to your body or your creative essence.

**Closing:** Read aloud the last paragraph of chapter 2 (page 82), and then close with a Circle Blessing.

## Session 3: Identity

**Readings:** Chapter 3: Embodying Your Womanhood
**Opening:** Read aloud the opening for chapter 3 (page 83) to call together the energy. Do a brief check-in for each woman.

**Group Discussion Questions:**

How do you embody your feminine identity?
Where have you given up your feminine ground and limited your expression of the feminine?
What is sacred to you, and how can this assist you in restoring your full feminine range?

**Group Reflection:** Have one woman lead the group in the Finding Your Root Voice exercise (page 95). Share your experiences and challenges in accessing the wisdom of your root and finding your own authentic feminine.

**Group Activity:** Do the Assessing Your Meaning of the Feminine exercise (page 85). Share your lists. Notice the similarities and differences in your perspectives. Reflect on the sacred feminine and speak your desires for new expressions of the feminine.

**Closing:** Read aloud the Body Blessing (page 123), and then close with a Circle Blessing.

## Session 4: Expression

**Readings:** Chapter 4: Expressing Your Wild Femininity
**Opening:** Read aloud the opening for chapter 4 (page 125) to call together the energy. Do a brief check-in for each woman.
**Group Discussion Questions:**

How do you experience the masculine/feminine divide?
Where in your life are you able to express and receive the warmth of your creative fire?
Where is your radiance diminished or your fire in need of tending?

**Group Reflection:** Have one woman lead the group in the Meditation on the Ovaries exercise (page 130). Notice which ovary you are more readily drawn to and how this is visible in your creative life. Share your discoveries and the wisdom received from your ovaries.

**Group Activity:** Look at the Daily Gestures for the Right and Left Ovaries exercise (page 167). Make a group list for cultivating your fire energy and making new masculine and feminine forms.

**Closing:** Read aloud the first paragraph of the Cultivate the Fire in Your Belly section (page 166), and then close with a Circle Blessing.

## Session 5: Fertility

**Readings:** Chapter 5: Returning to the Mother Place
**Opening:** Read aloud the opening for chapter 5 (page 179) to call together the energy. Do a brief check-in for each woman.
**Group Discussion Questions:**

What is fertility to you?
Where do you have a sense of abundance?
Where is there scarcity or a desire for more energy flow?

**Group Reflection:** Have one woman lead the Creative Essence Meditation (page 185). Share your reflections, present gestations, womb wisdom, or dreams for your creative essence.
**Group Activity:** Do the Redefining *Mother* exercise (page 183) as a group. Ponder your collective experience with the word *mother* and your creative potential as women.
**Closing:** Read aloud the last paragraph of chapter 5 (page 224), and then close with a Circle Blessing.

## Session 6: Lineage

**Readings:** Chapter 6: Transforming Your Inheritance
**Opening:** Read aloud the opening for chapter 6 (page 225) to call together the energy. Do a brief check-in for each woman.
**Group Discussion Questions:**

What do you know about your lineage that defines who you are?

Where is your lineage unknown, and what are you missing
  in its absence?
What other lines define your creative range?

**Group Reflection:** Have one woman lead the Lineage Meditation exercise (page 259). Share your experiences regarding the flow
of your mother and father lines.

**Group Activity:** Do the Name Your Fear exercise (page 237)
and share your discoveries. Discuss how your creative range would
change if you lived from a place of desire—with faith and trust—
rather than fear.

**Closing:** Read the Ancestor Blessing aloud (page 281), and then
close with a Circle Blessing.

## Session 7: Sacred Form

**Readings:** Chapter 7: Discovering Your Full Feminine Range
**Opening:** Read aloud the opening for chapter 7 (page 283) to
call together the energy. Do a brief check-in for each woman.
**Group Discussion Questions:**

What will you make as a woman?
Where have your forms (identities, relationships, creations,
  roles, ways of being, daily habits, body patterns, rituals,
  connections to spirit) become rigid rather than dynamic
  expressions?
How will you make new forms that embody the fullness of
  your womanhood and cultivate your joy?

**Group Reflection:** Have one woman lead the group in the
Opening Your Senses exercise (page 289). Notice how your awareness and your overall presence changes when your senses are open.
**Group Activity:** Do the Making a Spiritual Bath exercise (page
325) as a group with a large collective bowl. Each woman places her

own flowers or leaves into the bowl, and then together, witness your collective creation. Bless yourself with this sacred water. Read aloud the Sacred Pelvic Bowl exercise (page 348); ponder your sacred center.

**Closing:** Read aloud Calling on the Elements (page 346), and then close with a Circle Blessing.

After the completion of your seven gatherings, plan a meal, ritual, or creative activity that you can do as a group to celebrate your journey with the wild feminine. Share your experience of this journey with one another. Let your discussion inspire new rituals, daily gestures, creative expressions, root medicine, and other ways to continue restoring the range of the wild feminine in your every-day life.

# List of Exercises

# Starting a Wild Feminine Practice

This is a practice to develop new physical forms and energy pathways that reinforce and give expression to your core radiance. With a regular practice, your creative energy will become more abundant and you will witness the effects of this flow in all areas of your life. Like any habit, these beneficial patterns are strengthened with use. Establishing a practice of vibrancy and balance in your center, you will also be able to call on these resources to manifest your creations or in times of challenge to navigate the turbulence with grace.

### Physical Flow—Awaken the potential in your body

Daily: Attend to the needs of your body—movement, nourishment, rest, touch. Let your body guide you toward joy.

Weekly: Revitalize your center with a one-minute vaginal massage exercise in the shower (see page 368). Reduce sources of tension-causing stress, address emotional health.

Monthly: Do a longer vaginal massage, receive a holistic type of bodywork, make pleasure a priority.

### Energetic Flow—Invite vibrant energy to flow through your center

Daily: Practice pelvic mindfulness—be aware of the energy in your bowl. Let energy from your center inspire your outer direction—from simply organizing your day to making grand plans.

Weekly: Use pelvic organ energies to clear your center as needed, restore core balance and flow, and practice holding your desired intentions. Make room for what enlivens your energy; release what no longer inspires.

Monthly: Develop a creative practice as a way of living. Find ways to be more creative in all aspects of life.

**Spiritual Flow—Embody your radiance**
Daily: Invite the blessing of spirit with a one-minute meditation (see page 369). Let in love; give expression to your beauty.

Weekly: Make a spiritual bath (page 325); bless yourself and others on a regular basis.

Monthly: Connect with the deeper energy currents—go to a wild place, do lineage work, create a ritual.

We often cannot control experiences we may encounter, but we can choose our energy response. In periods of stress, conflict, or even confusion regarding our creative direction, there is a tendency to contract—increasing tension in the body and decreasing core energy flow. If instead we remember to focus on expansion—rather than contraction—we remain open to the greater energies that can be of assistance and change patterns that otherwise perpetuate scarcity. Replacing worry with prayer, fear with faith, shame with blessings, grief with peace, anger with love, we open ourselves to spirit—in the body, the breath, and the flow of life.

### One-Minute Vaginal Massage—Revitalize Your Center

1. Place a finger into the vagina. Touch the right side of your pelvic muscles and exhale with the intention: *I release anything I no longer need.*

2. Touch the left side of your pelvic muscles and exhale again with the intention: *I release anything I no longer need.*

3. Touch the right side of your pelvic muscles and breathe toward your right ovary: *I invite the radiance of my right ovary to fill my pelvic bowl.*

4. Touch the left side of your pelvic muscles and breathe toward your left ovary: *I invite the radiance of my left ovary to fill my pelvic bowl.*

5. Place your finger in the center of your vagina. Breathe toward this center of your bowl three times with these affirmations: *I am sacred; I am radiant; I bring my radiance to life.*

### One-Minute Meditation — Invite the Blessing of Spirit

This mediation can be done in silence, prayer, walking, or any activity. I often do this as a moving mediation while cleaning my house or beginning a project where I would like divine assistance.

1. Bring awareness to the center of your body.

2. Make a connection between the base of your pelvic bowl and the earth.

3. Make a connection between the crown of your head and the sky.

4. Imagine the life-giving energies of the earth and the sky flowing into your body and out from your center, expanding your potential as you sit, walk, create, or work on the task at hand. The energy blessing of spirit is always available to you when you move this creative energy through your center.

# Resources for Finding a Pelvic Care Practitioner

There are many ways to assist your personal practice, including finding a pelvic care practioner.

- Visit www.wildfeminine.com to find out more information about my own practice of Holistic Pelvic Care as well as a growing list of Holistic Pelvic Care providers.
- Call your local physical therapy clinic to inquire about a Women's Health Physical Therapist on staff. Interview any potential providers: Ask if they use vaginal massage in their treatment practice (because not all women's health physical therapists are trained in internal techniques). Ask about the types of pelvic conditions they treat. Those practitioners who treat pelvic pain (as opposed to just incontinence) often have the most advanced manual (hands-on) skills.
- Find a local practitioner of the Arvigo Techniques of Maya Massage. This technique, developed by naprapathic physician and herbalist Dr. Rosita Arvigo and based on traditional healing methods of Maya medicine, addresses pelvic flow and organ alignment through abdominal and sacral massage, for both women and men.
- Through the Barral Institute, find a local practitioner trained in abdominal or pelvic visceral massage (massage of the abdominal or pelvic organs). These techniques, developed by French osteopath Dr. Jean-Pierre Barral, also address core alignment and flow for both women and men.

*Take good care of your sacred center.*
*May the beauty shine—*
*May the bowl sing.*